Philosophy of Osteopathy

Andrew T. Still

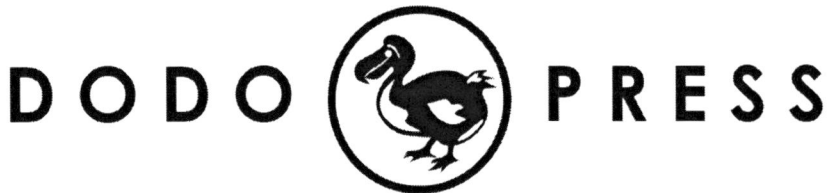

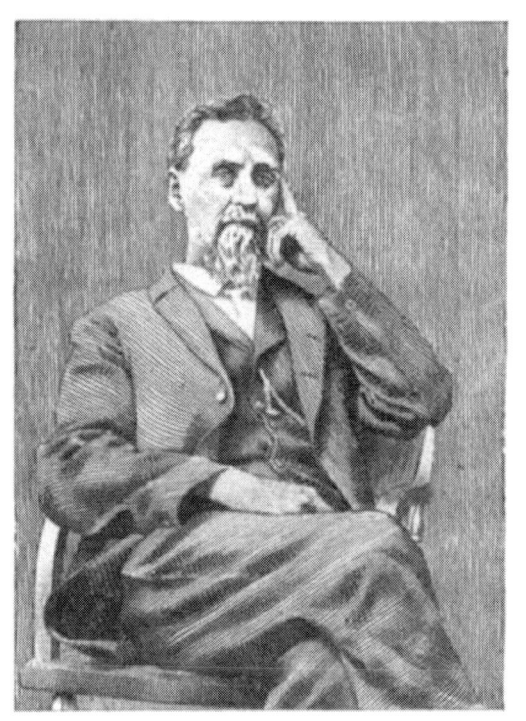

A. T. Still.

Philosophy of Osteopathy;

BY

ANDREW T. STILL,

DISCOVERER OF THE SCIENCE OF OSTEOPATHY AND
PRESIDENT OF THE AMERICAN SCHOOL
OF OSTEOPATHY.

1899.

PREFACE.

Many of my friends have been anxious ever since Osteopathy became an established fact, that I should write a treatise on the science. But I was never convinced that the time was ripe for such a production, nor am I even now convinced that this is not a little premature. Osteopathy is only in its infancy, it is a great unknown sea just discovered, and as yet we are only acquainted with its shore-tide.

When I saw others who had not more than skimmed the surface of the science, taking up the pen to write books on Osteopathy, and after having carefully examined their productions, found they were drinking from the fountains of old schools of drugs, dragging back the science to the very systems from which I divorced myself so many years ago, and realized that hungry students were ready to swallow such mental poison, dangerous as it was, I became fully awakened to the necessity of some sort of Osteopathic literature for those wishing to be informed.

This book is free from quotations from medical authors, and differs from them in opinion on almost every important question. I do not expect it to meet their approval; such a thing would be unnatural and impossible.

It is my object in this work to teach principles as I understand them, and not rules. I do not instruct the student to punch or pull a certain bone, nerve or muscle for a certain disease, but by a knowledge of the normal and abnormal, I hope to give a specific knowledge for all diseases.

This work has been written a little at a time for several years, just as I could snatch a moment from other cares to devote to it. I have carefully compiled these thoughts into a treatise. Every principle herein laid down has been fairly well tested by myself, and proven true.

The book has been written by myself in my own way, without any ambition to fine writing, but to give to the world a start in a philosophy that may be a guide in the future.

Owing to the great haste with which the book has been rushed through the press to meet the urgent demand, we will ask the indulgence of the public for any imperfection that may appear. Hoping the world may profit by these thoughts, I am,

Respectfully,
A. T. STILL.
Kirksville, Mo., Sept. 1, 1899.

CONTENTS.

CHAPTER VIII.
LIVER, BOWELS AND KIDNEYS.

Gender of the Liver—Productions of the Liver—A Hope for the Afflicted—Evidences of Truth—Loaded With Ignorance—Lack of Knowledge of the Kidney—How a Purgative Acts—Flux—Bloody Dysentery—Flux More Fully Described—Osteopathic Remedies—Medical Remedies—More of the Osteopathic Remedy.

CHAPTER IX.
THE BLOOD.

Uses for Fluids—Blood an Unknown Fluid—Harvey Only Reached the Banks of the River of Life—Blood Is Systematically Furnished—Fatality of Ignorance—To Find the Cause Must Be Honest—Following Arteries and Nerves—Feeding the Nerves—The Blood on Its Journey—Powers Necessary to Move Blood—Venous Blood Suspended.

CHAPTER X.
THE FASCIA.

Where Is Disease Sown?—An Illustration of Conception—The Greatest Problem—A Fountain of Supply—Fascia Omnipresent—Connection with Spinal Cord—Goes With and Covers All Muscles—Proofs in Contagion—Study of Nerves and Fascia—Tumefy—Tumefaction.

CHAPTER XI.
FEVERS.

Be Armed With Facts—Union of Human Gases With Oxygen—Fever and Nettle-rash. Nature Constructs for a Wise Purpose—Processes of Life Must be Kept in Motion—No Satisfaction from Authors—Animal Heat—Semeiology—Symptomatology—Definition of Fever—Fevers only Effects—Result of Stoppages of Vein or Artery—Aneurisms.

CHAPTER I.

SOME INTRODUCTORY REMARKS.

Not a Work of Compilation—Authors Quoted—Method of Reasoning—The Osteopath an Artist—When I Became an Osteopath—Dr. Neal's Opinion—The Opinions of Others—What Studies Necessary—What I Mean by Anatomy—Principles—The Practicing Osteopath's Guide—The Fascia—Not a Pleasing Task— Without Accepted Theories—Truths of Nature—Body, Motion and Mind—Osteopathy to Cure Disease—The Osteopath Should Find Health.

NOT A WORK OF COMPILATION.

To readers of my book on the Philosophy of Osteopathy, I wish to say that I will not tire you with a book of compilations just to sell to the anxious reader. As I have spent thirty years of my life reading and following rules and remedies used for curing, and learned in sorrow it was useless to listen to their claims, for instead of getting good, I obtained much harm therefrom, I asked for, and obtained a mental divorce from them, and I want it to be understood that drugs and I are as far apart as the East is from the West; now, and forever. Henceforth I will follow the dictates of nature in all I say or write.

AUTHORS QUOTED.

I quote no authors but God and experience when I write, or lecture to the classes or the masses, because no book written by medical writers can be of much use to us, and it would be very foolish to look to them for advice and instruction on a science they know nothing of. They are illy able to advise for themselves, they have never been asked to advise us, and I am free to say but few persons who have been pupils of my school have tried to get wisdom from medical writers and apply it as worthy to be taught as any part of Osteopathy, philosophy or practice. Several books have been compiled, called "Principles of Osteopathy." They may sell but will fail to give the knowledge the student desires.

METHOD OF REASONING.

The student of any philosophy succeeds best by the more simple methods of reasoning. We reason for needed knowledge only, and should try and start out with as many known facts as possible. If we would reason on diseases of the organs of the head, neck, abdomen or pelvis, we must first know where these organs are, how and from what arteries the eye, ear, or tongue is fed.

THE OSTEOPATH AN ARTIST.

I believe you are taught anatomy in our school more thoroughly than any other school to date, because we want you to carry a living picture of all or any part of the body in your mind as a ready painter carries the picture of the face, scenery, beast or any thing he wishes to represent by his brush. He would only be a waster of time and paint and make a daub that would disgust any one who would employ him. We teach you anatomy in all its branches, that you may be able to have and keep a living picture before your mind all the time, so you can see all joints, ligaments, muscles, glands, arteries, veins, lymphatics, fascia superficial and deep, all organs, how they are fed, what they must do, and why they are expected to do a part, and what would follow in case that part was not done well and on time. I feel free to say to my students, keep your minds full of pictures of the normal body all the time, while treating the afflicted.

WHEN I BECAME AN OSTEOPATH.

In answer to the questions of how long have you been teaching this discovery, and what books are essential to the study? I will say I began to give reasons for my faith in the laws of life as given to men, worlds and beings by the God of nature, June, 1874, when I began to talk and propound questions to men of learning. I thought the sword and cannons of nature were pointed and trained upon our systems of drug doctoring.

DR. NEAL'S OPINION.

I asked Dr. J. M. Neal, of Edinburg, Scotland, for some information that I needed badly. He was a medical doctor of five years training, a man of much mental ability, who would give his opinions freely and to the point. I have been told by one or more Scotch M. D.'s that a Dr. John M. Neal, of Edinburg, was hung for murder. He was not hung while with me. The only thing made me doubt him being a Scotchman was he loved whiskey, and I had been told that the Scotch were a sensible people. John M. Neal said that "drugs was the bait of fools"; it was no science, and the system of drugs was only a trade, followed by the doctor for the money that could be obtained by it from the ignorant sick. He believed that nature was a law capable of vindicating its power all over the world.

THE OPINIONS OF OTHERS.

As this writing is for the information of the student I will continue the history by saying, that in the early days of Osteopathy I sought the opinions of the most learned, such as Dr. Schnebly, Professor of Language and History in the Baker University, Baldwin, Kansas; Dr. Dallas, a very learned M. D. of the Alopathic faith; Dr. F. A. Grove, well-known in Kirksville; J. B. Abbott, Indian agent, and many others of renown. Then back to the tombs of the dead, to better acquaint myself with the systems of medicine and the foundations of truth upon which they stood, if any. I will not worry your patience with a list of the names of authors that have written upon the subject of medicine, as remedial agents. I will use the word that the theologian often uses when asked whom Christ died for, the answer universally is, ALL. All intelligent medical writers say by word or inference that drugs or drugging is a system of blind guess work, and if we should let our opinions be governed by the marble lambs and other emblems of dead babies found in the cemeteries of the world, we would say that John M. Neal was possibly hung for murder, not through design, but through traditional ignorance of the power of nature to cure both old and young, by skillfully adjusting the engines of life so as to bring forth pure and healthy blood, the greatest known germicide, to one capable to reason who has the skill to conduct the vitalizing and protecting fluids to throat, lungs and all parts of the system, and ward off diseases as nature's God has indicated. With this faith and method of reasoning, I began to treat diseases by Osteopathy as an experimenter, and notwithstanding I obtained good results in all cases in diseases of climate and contagions, I hesitated for years to proclaim to the world that there was but little excuse for a master engineer to lose a child in cases of diphtheria, croup, measles, mumps, whooping cough, flux and other forms of summer diseases, peculiar to children. Neither was it necessary for the adult to die with diseases of summer, fall and winter. But at last I took my stand on this rock and my confidence in nature, where I have stood and fought the battles, and taken the enemy's flag in every engagement for the last twenty-five years.

WHAT STUDIES NECESSARY.

As you contemplate studying this science and have asked to know the necessary studies, I wish to impress it upon your minds that you begin with anatomy, and you end with anatomy, a knowledge of anatomy is all you want or need, as it is all you can use or ever will use in your practice, although you may live one hundred years. You have asked for my opinion as the founder of the science. Yours is an honest question, and God being my judge I will give you just as honest an answer. As I have said, a knowledge of anatomy with its application covers every inch of ground that is necessary to qualify you to become a skillful and successful Osteopath, when you go forth into the world to combat diseases.

WHAT I MEAN BY ANATOMY.

I will now define what I mean by anatomy. I speak by comparison and tell you what belongs to the study of anatomy. I will take a chicken whose parts and habits all persons are familiar with to illustrate. The chicken has a head, a neck, a breast, a tail, two legs, two wings, two eyes, two ears, two feet, one gizzard, one crop, one set of bowels, one liver, and one heart. This chicken has a nervous system, a glandular system, a muscular system, a system of lungs and other parts and principles not necessary to speak of in detail. But

I want to emphasize, they belong to the chicken, and it would not be a chicken without every part or principle. These must all be present and answer roll call or we do not have a complete chicken. Now I will try and give you the parts of anatomy and the books that pertain to the same. You want some standard author on descriptive anatomy in which you learn the form and places of all bones, the place and uses of ligaments, muscles and all that belong to the soft parts. Then from the descriptive anatomy you are conducted into the dissecting room, in which you receive demonstrations, and are shown all parts through which blood and other fluids are conducted. So far you see you are in anatomy. From the demonstrator you are conducted to another room or branch of anatomy called physiology, a knowledge of which no Osteopath can do without and be a success. In that room you are taught how the blood and other fluids of life are produced, and the channels through which this fluid is conducted to the heart and lungs for purity and other qualifying processes, previous to entering the heart for general circulation to nourish and sustain the whole human body. I want to insist and impress it upon your minds that this is as much a part of anatomy as a wing is a part of a chicken. From this room of anatomy you are conducted to the room of histology, in which the eye is aided by powerful microscopes and made acquainted with the smallest arteries of the human body, which in life are of the greatest known importance, remembering that in the room of histology you are still studying anatomy, and what that machinery can and does execute every day, hour, and minute of life. From the histological room you are conducted to the room of elementary chemistry, in which you learn something of the laws of association of substances, that you can the better understand what has been told you in the physiological room, which is only a branch of anatomy, and intended to show you that nature can and does successfully compound and combine elements for muscles, blood, teeth and bone. From there you are taken to the room of the clinics, where you are first made acquainted with both the normal and abnormal human body, which is only a continuation of the study of anatomy. From there you are taken to the engineer's room (or operator's room) in which you are taught how to observe and detect abnormalities and the effect or effects they may and do produce, and how they effect health and cause that condition known as disease.

PRINCIPLES.

Principles to an Osteopath means a perfect plan and specification to build in form a house, an engine, a man, a world, or anything for an object or purpose. To comprehend this engine of life or man which is so constructed with all conveniences for which it was made, it is necessary to constantly keep the plan and specification before the mind, and in the mind, to such a degree that there is no lack of knowledge of the bearings and uses of all parts. After a complete knowledge of all parts with their forms, sizes and places of attachment which should be so thoroughly grounded in the memory that there would be no doubt of the intent of the builder for the use or purpose of the great and small parts, and why they have a part to perform in the workings of the engine. When this part of the specification is thoroughly learned from anatomy or the engineer's guide book, he will then take up the chapter on the division of forces, by which this engine moves and performs the duties for which it was created. In this chapter the mind will be referred to the brain to obtain a knowledge of that organ, where the force starts, how it is conducted to any belt, pully, journal, or division of the whole building. After learning where the force is obtained, and how conveyed from place to place throughout the whole body, he becomes interested and wisely instructed. He sees the various parts of this great system of life when preparing fluids commonly known as blood, passing through a set of tubes both great and small—some so vastly small, as to require the aid of powerful microscopes to see their infinitely small forms, through which the blood and other fluids are conducted by the heart and force of the brain, to construct organs, muscles, membranes and all the things necessary to life and motion, to the parts separately and combined. By this minute acquaintance with the normal body which has been learned in the specification as written in standard authors of anatomy and the dissecting rooms, he is well prepared to be invited into the inspection room to receive comparisons between the normal and abnormal engines, built according to nature's plan and specification, and absolutely perfect. He is called into this room for the purpose of comparing engines that have been strained from being thrown off the track, or run against other bodies with such force as to bend journals, pipes, break or loosen bolts; or otherwise deranged, so as to render it useless until repaired. To repair signifies to readjust from the abnormal condition in which the machinist finds it, to the condition of the normal engines which stand in the shop of repairs. His inspection would commence by first lining up the wheels with straight journals; then he would naturally be conducted to the boiler, steam chest, shafts, and every part that belongs to a completed engine. To know that they are straight and in place as shown upon the plan and described by the specification, he has done all that is required of a master mechanic. Then it goes into the hands of the engineer, who waters, fires and conducts this artificial being on its journey. You as Osteopathic machinists can go no farther than to adjust the abnormal condition, in which you find the afflicted. Nature will do the rest.

THE PRACTICING OSTEOPATH'S GUIDE.

The Osteopath reasons if he reasons at all, that order and health are inseparable, and that when order in all parts is found, disease cannot prevail, and if order is complete and disease should be found, there is no use for order. And if order and health are universally one in union, then the doctor cannot usefully, physiologically, or philosophically be guided by any scale of reason, otherwise. Does a chemist get results desired by accident? Are your accidents more likely to get good results than his? Does order and success demand thought and cool headed reason? If we wish to be governed by reason, we must take a position that is founded on truth and capable of presenting facts, to prove the validity of all truths we present. A truth is only a hopeful supposition if it is not supported by results. Thus all nature is kind enough to willingly exhibit specimens of its work as vindicating witnesses of its ability to prove its assertions by its work. Without that tangible proof, nature would belong to the gods of chance. The laws of mother, conception, growth and birth, from atoms to worlds would be a failure, a universe without a head to direct. But as the beautiful works of nature stand to-day, and in all time past, fully able by the evidence it holds before the eye and mind of reason, that all beings great and small came by the law of cause and effect, are we not bound to work by the laws of cause, if we wish an effect? If the heavens do move by cause when was its beings divorced from that great common law? Are we not bound to trust and work by the old and reliable self-evident laws, until something later has proven its superior ability to ward off disease and cure the sick.

THE FASCIA.

I know of no part of the body that equals the fascia as a hunting ground. I believe that more rich golden thought will appear to the mind's eye as the study of the fascia is pursued than any division of the body. Still one part is just as great and useful as any other in its place. No part can be dispensed with. But the fascia is the ground in which all causes of death do the destruction of life. Every view we take, a wonder appears. Here we find a place for the white corpuscles building anew and giving strength to throw impurities from the body by tubes that run from the skin to tanks of useful fluids, that would heap up and are no longer of use in the body. No doubt nerves exist in the fascia, that change the fluid to gas, and force it through the spongy and porous system as a delivery by the vital chain of wonders, that go on all the time to keep nerves wholly pure.

NOT A PLEASANT TASK.

I dislike to write, and only do so, when I think my productions will go into the hands of kind-hearted geniuses who read, not to find a book of quotations, but to go with the soul of the subject that is being explored for its merits,—weigh all truths and help bring its uses front for the good of man.

Osteopathy has not asked a place in written literature prior to this date, and does not hope to appear on written pages even to suit the author of this imperfectly written book.

WITHOUT ACCEPTED THEORIES.

Columbus had to launch and navigate much and long, and meet many storms, because he had not the written experience of other travelers to guide him. He had only a few bits of drift-wood not common to his home growth, to cause him to move as he did. But there was a fact, a bit of wood that did not grow on his home soil.

He reasoned that it must be from some land amid the sea whose shores had not before been known to his race. With these facts and his powerful mind of reason, he met all opposition, and moved alone; just as all men do who have no use for theories as their compass to guide them through the storms. This opposition a mental explorer must meet.

I felt that I must anchor my boat to living truths and follow them wheresoever they might drift. Thus I launched my boat many years ago on the open seas, fearlessly, and have never found a wave of scorn nor abuse that truth could not eat, and do well on.

TRUTHS OF NATURE.

We often speak of truth. We say great truths, and use many other qualifying expressions. But no one truth is greater than any other truth. Each has a sphere of usefulness peculiar to itself. Thus we should treat with respect and reverence all truths, great and small. A truth is the complete work of nature, which can only be demonstrated by the vital principle belonging to that class of truths. Each truth or division as we see it, can only be made known to us by the self evident fact, which this truth is able to demonstrate by its action.

If we take man as our object to base the beginning of our reason, we find the association of many elements, which differ in kind to suit the purpose for which they were designed. To us they act, to us they are wisely formed and located for the purpose for which they were designed. Through our five senses we deal with the material body. It has action. That we observe by vision which connects the mind to reason. High above the five senses on the subject of cause or causes of this, is motion. By the testimony of the witness the mind is connected in a manner by which it can reason on solidity and size. By smell, taste and sound, we make other connections between the chambers of reason and the object we desire to reason upon; and thus our foundation on which all five witnesses are arrayed to the superior principle which is mind.

After seeing a human being complete in form, self moving, with power to stop or go on at will, to us he seems to obey some commander. He seems to go so far and stop; he lies down and gets up; he turns round and faces the objects that are traveling in the same direction he does. Possibly he faces the object by his own action. Then by about facing, he sees one coming with greater velocity, sees he can not escape by his own speed, so he steps aside and lets that body pass on, as though he moved in obedience to some order. The bystander would ask the question, "How did he know such a dangerous body was approaching?" He finds on the most crucial examination, that the sense of hearing is wholly without reason. The same is true with all the five senses pertaining to man, beast, or bird. This being the condition of the five physical senses, we are forced by reason to conclude there is a superior being who conducts the material man, sustains, supports and guards against danger; and after all our explorations, we have to decide that man is triune when complete.

BODY, MOTION AND MIND.

First the material body, second the spiritual being, third a being of mind which is far superior to all vital motions and material forms, whose duty is to wisely manage this great engine of life. This great principle known as mind, must depend for all evidences on the five senses, and on this testimony, all mental conclusions are bad, and all orders from this mental court are issued to move to any point or stop at any place. Thus to obtain good results, we must blend ourselves with, and travel in harmony with nature's truths. When this great machine man, ceases to move in all its parts, which we call death, the explorers knife discovers no mind, no motion. He simply finds formulated matter with no motor to move it, with no mind to direct it. He can trace the channels through which the fluids have circulated, he can find the relation of parts to other parts; in fact by the knife, he can expose to view the whole machinery that once was wisely active. Suppose the explorer is able to add the one principle motion, at once we would see an action, but it would be a confused action. Still he is not the man desired to be produced. There is one addition that is indispensable to control this active body, or machine, and that is mind. With that added the whole machinery then works as man. The three when united in full action are able to exhibit the thing desired—complete.

OSTEOPATHY TO CURE DISEASE.

The Osteopath seeks first physiological perfection of form, by normally adjusting the osseous frame work, so that all arteries may deliver blood to nourish and construct all parts. Also that the veins may carry away all impurities dependent upon them for renovation. Also that the nerves of all classes may be free and unobstructed while applying the powers of life and motion to all divisions, and the whole system of nature's laboratory.

A full and complete supply of arterial blood must be generated and delivered to all parts, organs and glands, by the channels called the arteries. And when it has done its work, then without delay the veins must return all to heart and lungs for renewal. We must know some delay of fluids has been established on which nature begins the work of renewal by increased action of electricity, even to the solvent action of fever heat, by which watery substances evaporate and relieve the lymphatic system of stagnant, watery secretions. Thus fever is a natural and powerful remedy.

THE OSTEOPATH SHOULD FIND HEALTH.

To find health should be the object of the doctor. Anyone can find disease. He should make the grand round among the sentinels and ascertain if they are asleep, dead or have deserted their posts, and have allowed the enemy to get into camps. He should visit all posts. Before he goes out to make the rounds, he should know where all posts are, and the value of the supply he has charge of, whether it be shot, shell, grub, clothing, arms or anything of value to the Company or Division.

CHAPTER II.

Osteopathic Explorations.

Divisions of the Body—Searching for the Cause—Duty of the Osteopathic Explorer—Classification and Division—The Abnormal—Nerve Powers—Witnesses to Examine—Abnormal Growths—Cerebro Spinal Fluid—Body in Perfect Health—Chemistry—Nature's Chemistry.

DIVISIONS OF THE BODY.

After many long years, treating and trying to teach the student of Osteopathy how to hunt for and find the local causes of diseases, not contagious, or infectious, I have succeeded in planning and suggesting a method, which I am sure the doctor can easily follow, and find any diversion from the normal, that would interfere with the nerves, veins, and arteries, of any organ or limb of the body. I have formulated a simple mental diagram that divides the body into three parts, chest, upper and lower limbs. The first division takes in head, neck, chest, abdomen and pelvis. The second division takes in head, neck, lower and upper arm and hand. The third division takes in foot, leg, thigh, pelvis and lumbar vertebra. I make this division for the purpose of holding the explorer to the limits of all supplies. In the ellipse of the chest is found all vital supplies; then from that center of life we have two branches only, one of the arm, and one of the lower limb. In each division we have five points of exploration.[1]

SEARCHING FOR THE CAUSE.

To illustrate, we will take the lower limb, whether there is lameness, soreness, gouty, rheumatic, neuralgic, swollen, shrunken, feverish, cold, smooth and glassy, sores, ulcers, erysipelas, milkleg, varicose veins, or any defect that the patient may complain of, who is the only reliable book or being of symptomatology. For convenience we will divide that lower limb into five parts, the foot, leg, thigh, pelvis and lumbar region. The patient (symptomatologist) tells us he has a pain in front, center and under part of foot. Now the doctor or bird dog, can find quails of reason in but one field that would lead him to the cause. As this field is divided into five parts and the hunter has carefully searched four divisions, he will find the cause or causes in the fifth and none other. If a dislocated bone is not found in the foot after ascertaining that there has been no crushing by falling bodies, horses feet, stepping on glass, nails and other things that would penetrate the foot, and irritate by being broken off, closed and remaining in the flesh; we will explore the leg for the quail, ascertain if the articulation is normal at ankle and knee. If we find the bone is not broken, the leg has no splinters of wood, nor injured flesh by bites from dogs or other animals, nor any other substance that would injure the leg, we are prepared to pass on and explore another place for pain in the foot. We go on to division No. 3 or the thigh division, and ascertain if the thigh is normal in all conditions, properly in socket, with all muscles, ligaments and nerves unoppressed. There are but two more divisions left for exploration, and they are the most important and interesting of the five, the pelvis and lumbar, through which all the nerves of the limb pass. We must stop at pelvis and observe carefully that there is no twist of ligaments before going to lumbar, which is the last of the five divisions. If we have found nothing in the previous four, and have explored them as carefully as we should, we have but one brush heap left, and that one contains the quail that we have been hunting for. As the lumbar contains and conveys all nerve forces to the pelvis from the brain and all divisions of the lower limbs, we will now examine the articulations of that part of the spine, and in that we are very certain to find the cause if we have made no mistake in our examination in the preceding divisions of the limb. As we enter the exploration of this part of the spine we must remember that we are about to deal with the many divisions of the nerves of the *cauda equina*. The great question before us, comes after this form. What would wound or bruise any division of nerves that would lead by the way of the great or lesser sciatic, to a bone in the front and under side of the foot? Jars, strains, twists, and dislocations, must be carefully searched for. A partial dislocation of one side of the spine would produce a twist which would throw one muscle on to another and another, straining ligaments, producing conjestion and inflammation, or some irritation that would lead to a suspension of the fluids necessary to the harmonious vitality of the foot, which is the great and only cause by which the suffering is produced in a foreign land, which we call a famine in the foot.

DUTY OF THE OSTEOPATHIC EXPLORER.

This method of exploration is not directed by the sound of the fog-horns of unreliable and unsatisfactory symptomatology. Osteopathy has a method of its own, which is correct or it has no method at all, and is guided by the surveyor's compass that will find all corners as established by the orders of the government and surveyor's general. Thus an Osteopath must find the true corners as set by the Divine Surveyor. The general surveyor hands our plats and specifications to the division general, with instructions to establish all lines and divisions, state, county, township and sections, and mark each one by stones or otherwise, so they cannot be lost; but are findable by any competent surveyor who follows the field notes displayed in anatomy. Thus you would see a successful Osteopath is guided by the field notes of nature to all corners, his business is to know that every corner stone is in its place, standing erect as nature designed and established it. If he tolerates any variation of this stone or stones from the place or places that God the grand surveyor of the universe has placed them, he will observe there is an infringement and cause for inharmony and discord of the possessors of the four quarter sections of land, for which this cornerstone was placed; and his sworn duty is to bring this stone from any variation from the field notes and establish it where it was first placed. Thus his ability to find the true corners and adjust all stones will mark him as a successful Osteopath.

CLASSIFICATION AND DIVISION.

I will classify or divide man's body for convenience of exploration for diseases into head and neck first; then head, neck and chest, third, head, neck, chest and abdomen; then unite head, neck, chest, abdomen and sacrum. I will take up a few diseases under each division as they are located. By this method I think I can better show what nerves should be more or less active.

THE ABNORMAL.

A lesion may and does appear on a part or all of the person which may appear as a growth or withering away of a limb in all its muscles, nerves and blood supply. As in case of tumors on scalp, loss of hair, eruptions of face, growth of tonsils, ulcers of one or both ears, growths on outside and inside of eyes, a cause must precede an effect in all cases. A pain in head is an effect; cause is older than the effect and is absolute in all variations from normal conditions. A tumor on the head and under the skin is an effect only. It took matter to give it size, it took power to deliver that substance, the fact that a tumor was formed, shows that the power to build was present and did the work of construction. Another power should have been there to complete the work at that location; that power is the offbearing of the dead matter after the work of construction was complete.

NERVE POWERS.

If we think as men of reason should, we will count five nerve powers. They must all be present to build a part, and must answer promptly at roll call and work all the time. The names of these master workmen are sensation, motion, nutrition, voluntary and involuntary. All must answer at every roll call during life; none can be granted a leave of absence for a moment. Suppose sensation should leave a limb for a time, have we not a giving away of all cells and glands? An undue filling up follows quickly because sensation limits and tells when the supply is too great for the use of the builder's purpose. Suppose the nerve power known as motion should fail for a time, starvation would soon begin its deadly work for want of food. Suppose again the nerves of nutrition should fail to apply the nourishing showers we would surely die in sight of food. With the voluntary nerves we move or stay at the will of he or she who wishes to give direction to the motor powers, at any time a change by action is required. At this time I will stop defining the several and varied uses of the five kinds of nerves, and begin to account for growths and other variations, from the healthy to the unhealthy conditions of man. The above named are the five known powers of animal life, and to direct them wisely is the work of the doctor of Osteopathy.

WITNESSES TO EXAMINE.

He has five witnesses to examine in all cases he has under his care. He must give close attention to the source and supply of healthy blood. If blood is too scant he must look to the motor systems of blood making, that would surely invite his most careful attention and study of the abdomen. He cannot expect blood to quietly pass through the diaphragm if impeded by muscular constriction around aorta, vena cava or thoracic duct. The diaphragm can and is often pulled down on both vena cava and thoracic duct, obstructing blood and chyle from returning to heart so much as to limit the chyle below the requirement of healthy blood, or even suppress the nerve action of lymphatics to such degree as to cause dropsy of the abdomen, or a stoppage of venous blood by pressure on vena cava so long that venous blood would be in stages of ferment when it enters the heart for renovation, and when purified and returned the supply is too small to sustain life to a normal standard.

ABNORMAL GROWTHS.

Thus the importance of a careful attention to the normal certainty of all the ribs to which the diaphragm is attached is essential. The eleventh and twelfth ribs may, and do often get pushed so far from their normal bearings, that they are often found turned in a line with the spine, with cartilaginous ends down near ilio-lumbar articulation. When in such position they draw the diaphragm down heavily on vena cava at about the fourth lumbar. Then you have cause for intermittent pulse, as the heart finds no passage of blood through the prolapsed diaphragm which is also stopping the vena cava and producing universal stagnation of blood and other fluids in all organs and glands below the diaphragm. Thus you have a beginning for abnormal growths of womb, kidneys and all lymphatics of liver, kidneys, spleen, pancreas, and all tumors of abdomen.

CEREBRO SPINAL FLUID.

To satisfy the mind of a philosopher who is mentally capable of asking for and knowing truth, when presented by nature, you must come at him outside of the limits of conjecture, and address him with self-evident truths only. When he takes up the philosophy of the great subject of life, to him who does know truth, no substitute can to any degree satisfy his mental demands. To the one who would deal in conjectures or suppose so's, he will at once be placed in the proper category to which he belongs, which is the drift-wood that floats down the dark river that is overshadowed by the nightmare of ignorance and superstition. A seeker after truth, is a man of few words, and they are used by him only by the truths or facts discovered. He has no patience with the unmeaning records offered only to please the credulous, and by those of little or no truth that appears during a long recitation of ungrounded statements. From the above it is wisely seen that the object of these remarks is to present a few truths for the purpose of stimulating the attention of the listener. We will take man when formed. When we use the word formed, we mean the whole building being complete. The brain with all organs, nerves, vessels, and every minutia in form with all materials found or used in life.

BODY IN PERFECT HEALTH.

We look at it in perfect health which means perfection and harmony not in part, but of the whole body. So far we are only filled with love, wonder and admiration. Another period of observation appears to the philosopher. We find partial or universal discord from the lowest observable to the highest in action and death. Then the book of whys is opened and displays its leaves which calls out mental labor even to the degree of agony, to know the cause or causes that produce a failure of a limb in sensation, motion, nutrition, voluntary and involuntary functional exhibits. His mind will explore the bone, the ligament, the muscle, the fascia, the channels through which the blood travels from heart to local destiny, with lymphatics and their contents,—the nerves, the blood vessels and every channel through or over which all substances are transmitted all over the body, particularly the disabled limb in question. It proceeds too and does obtain blood abundantly to and from the heart, but the results obtained are not satisfactory, and another leaf is opened of why no good results are obtained and where is the mystery, what quality and element of force and vitality has been withheld? A thought strikes him that the cerebro spinal fluid is the highest known element that is contained in the human body, and unless the brain furnishes this fluid in abundance a disabled condition of the body will remain. He who is able to reason will see that this great river of life must be tapped and the withering field irrigated at once, or the harvest of health be forever lost.

CHEMISTRY.

As chemical compounds are not known to Osteopathy to be used as remedies, then its use as a study for the student is only to teach that elements in nature do combine and form other substances, and without changes and unions, no teeth, bone, hair, or muscle could appear in the body from the food eaten. Then chemistry is of great use as a part of a thorough Osteopathic education. It gives us the reasons why food is found in the body as bone, muscle and so on, to all kinds of flesh, teeth and bones found in animal forms. Unless we know chemistry reasonably well, we can not do away with much mental worry of what becomes of food after eating. By chemistry the truths of physiology are firmly established in the mind of the student of nature, that in man a chemistry of wonderful powers does all the work of animal forms, and that in the laboratory of nature's chemistry is the ruling power. By elementary chemistry we are led to see the beauties of physiology only. Thus chemistry of the elementary is one, and physiology is the witness that it is law in man as in all nature. Thus in chemistry we comprehend some of the laws of union in nature which we can use mentally with knowing confidence. In chemistry we become acquainted with the law of cause and change in union, which is a standard law sought by the student of Osteopathy.

NATURE'S CHEMISTRY.

Osteopathy believes that all parts of the human body do work on chemical compounds, and from the general supply manufacture for local wants; thus the liver builds for itself of the material that is prepared in its own division laboratory. The same of heart and brain. No disturbing or hindering causes will be tolerated to stay if an Osteopath can find and remove it. We must reason that to withhold the supply from a limb, to wither away would be natural. We suffer from two causes. First, want of supply (hunger), and the burdens of dead deposits along nerve centers, which five nerves by chemical changes while in fermentation should regulate local or general divisions.

CORRECT METHOD OF REASONING.

In concluding this chapter we will confine our labor to an effort to direct the beginner to a correct method of reasoning. When he is brought face to face with the stern realities of the "sick room," the Osteopath begins his inquiries and follows with his questions just far enough to know what division of the body is in trouble. If he finds an arm has lost motion, he goes to arm to explore for cause. He can begin his hunt for cause at hand, explore it carefully for wounds, strains or any lesion that could injure nerves of the arm. If he finds no probable cause there, he should explore bones for dislocations or strains of ligaments at elbow; if he finds no defect there sufficient to locate cause in lower arm or hand; he has only two more places left to inspect, the shoulder and neck with their articulations of bone and muscles. If found normal at shoulder, then go to neck, out of which go all or most of the nerves of the arm; if he finds no lesion or cause equal to the trouble so far, then he has been careless in his search and should go over and over from marrow to periostium of all bones of the neck and head, because there are only five divisions in which a lesion can exist. Carefully look, think, feel and know that the head of the humerus is true in the glenoid cavity, clavicle true at both ends of its articulation, with sternum and acromion processes. See that the biceps are in their grooves, and ribs on spine are true at manubrium and spine, and that neck is true on first dorsal. True in all joints of the neck, as the nerves of the arm come from the neck, there must be no variation from normal, or trouble will appear from that cause. As the neck has much to do with the arm, we should keep a living picture of the forms of each bone, how and where it articulates with others, how it is joined by ligaments, what blood vessels, nerves and muscles cross or range with it lengthwise, because to overlook a small nerve and blood vessel you may fail to remove a goitre, and all diseases of the head, face and neck.

CHAPTER III.

The Head.

A Free Circulation—Death Blows—Something of the Neck—Order
of Treatment—The Pelvis—Brains of Animals—Arterial Motion—
Mental Vibrations—Overburdening the Mind—Hemiplegia.

A FREE CIRCULATION.

Before we treat of the head, we must follow blood from the heart to
all organs of the head. Not only look at the pictures in Gray, Morris,
Gerrish, or some finely illustrated work on anatomy, but we must
apply a searching hand and know to a certainty that the constrictors
of neck, or other muscles or ligaments do not pull cervical and hyoid
bones so close as to bruise pneumogastric or any other nerves or
fibres that would cause spasmodic contraction of digastric, stylo-
hyoid or the whole remaining group of neck muscles and ligaments,
with which you are or should be very familiar. Ever remember that
the venous drainage must be kept normally active or congestion, and
tumefaction, with inflammation of the glands of the head, face and
neck will appear, and mark for you this oversight; because the
perpetual health, ease and comfort of the head beginning with the
scalp and hair, with their nerves, glands and purity of blood supply,
a healthy eye, good hearing, healthy action of brain with its magnetic
and electric forces to the vital parts which sustain life, memory and
reason, depend directly and wholly upon unlimited freedom of the
circulatory system of nerves, blood and cerebral fluid. They must be
normal in action and quantity unembarrassed, otherwise bad
hearing, ulcers of the ears, cross eyes, pterygium, cataract,
granulated lids, staphyloma, lachrymosis and up to full list of
diseases of the eye, with tonsilitis, injured voice, tumors and cancers
of face, head, tongue, mouth and throat, along with erysipelas,
blotches and pimples, and all diseases of the glandular system of the
head and neck. Undoubtedly all these afflictions have their origin in
obstructed normal action between the heart and the termination of
all above it, for want of nerve and blood harmony.

DEATH BLOWS.

Remember that death blows are dealt out freely above the sternum by irritation and constriction of the parts above described. We should often refresh our minds, beginning with the muscles that connect the head and neck, and know to a certainty as we explore that junction that the capitas minor, major and lateralis, long and short of both anticus and posticus regions are indisputably normal to your hand and judgment. It is almost useless to say to the anatomist who has had the drilling in all branches of that science, previous to obtaining his diploma, to commence and detail the venous and excretory system, through which all those glands are drained, and kept in a healthy condition, but we say this much; let your morning, noon and evening prayer be this, Oh Lord! give me more anatomy each day I live, because experience has taught me the unavoidable demands when in the "sick room."

SOMETHING OF THE NECK.

Before you leave that wisely constructed neck, I want to press and imprint on your minds in the strongest terms that the wisest anatomist, and physiologist, the oldest and most successful Osteopath knows only enough of the neck, and its wondrous system of nerves, blood and muscles and its relation to all above and below it, to say, "From everlasting to everlasting thou art great, O Lord God Almighty!" Thy wisdom is surely boundless, for I see that man must be wise to know all about the neck, for we find by a twist of neck, we may become blind, deaf, spasmodic, lose speech and memory, and all that is known as the joys of man. On that division of the body all action of arms, legs, chest and all muscles get their life—power and motion. Think for a moment of the thousands and tens of thousands of large and small fluid vessels that pass to and from heart and brain, to every organ, bone, fibre, muscle and gland, both large and small, receiving and appropriating the substances as prepared in the chemical laboratory; so wisely situated, and so exact in all its works in the production and application of all substances in the body.

ORDER OF TREATMENT.

The reader will begin with the brain or head because I want to start with the head; first give such diseases as belong to that division of the body. Then the neck, chest, abdomen and pelvis. Thus we have five divisions in regular order, beginning with the head and finishing with the sacrum. The reader will find diseases of eye, ear, tongue, nose, face, scalp and hair under the chapter treating of the head. Next in regular order will be the division of the neck, with diseases of tonsils and glands of neck, swallow, trachæ, nerves, blood vessels and muscles, fascia and lymphatics, superior cervical ganglion and other nerves of the neck, as they affect vitality in diseases. Then we pass on to third division, with diseases of lung, heart, pericardium, and pleura, with all parts of chest. Then abdomen, liver, stomach and bowels, and all organs with resisting power of diaphragm. Fifth, pelvis, with its great supply of nerves, blood and other fluids. These give us cause to halt and seat the mind for a long season of observation. A great field opens at this point for the observing thinker.

THE PELVIS.

In the pelvis we find a system of nerves and arteries with blood for local supply, besides blood to construct womb, bladder, rectum, colon, cellular system and all the muscles of that cavity (the pelvis) all of which comes from arteries and branches above. We think it is not necessary to name them only in bulk, to a student versed in anatomy. Perhaps less is known of the pelvic system and its functions than any division of the body, and for that reason I have felt that we should know all that is possible to be learned. I believe more ignorance prevails to-day of internal causes of diseases than would if we reasoned that the pelvic nerves and vessels had much to do in forming the abdominal viscera.

THE BRAIN OF ANIMALS.

Of all parts of the body of man to be well studied, the brain should be the most attractive. It is the place where all force centers, where all nerves connect to one common battery. By its orders the laboratory of life begins to move on crude material and labors until blood is formed and becomes food for all nerves first; then arteries and veins by nerve action and forces, to suit each class of work to be done by that set of nerves which is to construct forms; keep blood constantly in motion by the arteries and from all parts back to the heart, through the veins, that the blood may be purified, renewed and re-enter the arteries to be taken to all places of need.

ARTERIAL MOTION.

Arterial motion is normal during all ages, from the quick pulse of the babe's arm, to the ages of each year to one hundred or more. At this great age the pulse is so slow that the heat is not generated by the nerves, whose motor velocity is not great enough to bring electricity to the stage of heat. All heat, high and low, surely is the effect of active electricity—plus to fever; minus to coldness. When an irritant enters the body by lung, skin or any other way, a change appears in the heart's action from its effects on the brain, to the high electric action and that burning heat called fever. If plus violent type (yellow fever), if minus, low grades (typhus, typhoid, plagues), and so on through the list.

MENTAL VIBRATIONS.

To think implies action of the brain. We can grade thought although we cannot measure its speed.

Suppose a person of one kind of business thinks just fast enough to suit that profession. A man is engaged in raising hogs and that alone. He must reason on and of the nature of hogs. He begins about so: a hog eats, drinks, bathes, roots and sleeps. He knows the hog eats grain, so he feeds it corn, or some other suitable cereal, with plenty of water and good bedding. The swine is on his mind night and day.

THE WHEELS OF THOUGHT.

Now the question is, how fast does he think? How many revolutions do the wheels of his head make per minute to do all the necessary thinking connected with the hog business? Say his mental wheels revolve 100 times each minute. Then he adds sheep to his business, and if that should require 100 more revolutions and he takes charge of raising draft horses with 175 revolutions added, you see the wheels of his head whizzing off 375 vibrations per minute. And at this time he adds the duties of the carpenter with 300 more revolutions, add them together and you see 675. To this number he adds the duties and thoughts of a sheriff, which are numerous enough to buzz his wheels at 1500 more, you find 2175 to be his mental revolutions so far. Now you have the great physical demands added to the mental motion which his brain has to support, yet he can do all so far, fairly well.

OVERBURDENING THE MIND.

He now adds to his labors the manufacturing of leather, from all kinds of hides, with the chemistry of fine tanning, which is equal to all previous mental motions. Add and you find 4250 revolutions all drawing on his brain each minute of the day. Add to this mental strain the increased action of his body which has to perform these duties and you see the beginning of a worry of both mind and body, to which you add manufacturing of engines, iron puddling, rolling, etc.; a delegate to a national convention, thoughts of the death of a near relative; add to this a security debt to meet during a money panic. By this time the mind begins to fag below the power of resistance.

HEMIPLEGIA.

Duration of such great mental vibrations for so long stops nutrition of all or one-half of the brain, and we have a case of "Hemiplegia," or the wheels of one-half of the brain run so fast as to overcome some fountain of nerve force and explode some cerebral artery in the brain and deposit a clot of blood at some motor supply or plexus.

Thus we see men from over mental action fall in our National councils, courts, manufactories, churches, and almost all places of great mental activity. Slaves and savages seldom fall victims to paralysis of any kind, but escape all such, for they know nothing of the strains of mind and hurried nutrition. They eat and rest, live long and happy. The idea of riches never bothers their slumbers. Physical injuries may and often do wound motor, sensory and nutrient centers of brain; but the effect is just the same, partial or complete suspension of the motor and sensory systems.

If you burst a boiler by high pressure or otherwise, your engine ceases to move. And just the same of an over-worked brain or body.

Hemiplegia. "The half" and "I strike." Paralysis of one half of the body.[2]

Hemiplegia is usually the result of a cerebral hemorrhage or embolism. It sometimes occurs suddenly without other marked symptoms, but commonly it is ushered in by an apoplectic attack and on return of consciousness it is observed that one side of the body is paralyzed, the paralysis being often profound in the beginning, and disappearing to a greater or less extent at a later period.

Hemiplegia is much more rarely produced by a tumor. It then generally comes on slowly, the paralysis gradually increasing as the neoplasm encroaches more and more upon the motor tracks, though the tumor may be complicated by the occurrence of a hemorrhage and a sudden hemiplegia.

A gradual hemiplegia may also be produced by an abcess or chronic softening of the brain substance. Other conditions or symptoms presented, will in such case, assist us to diagnose the nature of the lesion.

CHAPTER IV.

Ear Wax and Its Uses.

Nature Makes Nothing in Vain—A Successful Experiment—A Question for Ages—The Position—Meaning of Life—Some Questions Asked—Condition in Certain Diseases Caused by Cold—Cerumen in Fluid State—Winter Kills Babies—Some Advice to Mothers—A Case in Point—Connection of the brain and Other Nerves in Digestion—Unaided Investigation.

NATURE MAKES NOTHING IN VAIN.

That nature makes nothing in vain is an established truth in the minds of all persons whose observation has created in such persons a desire to reason, and that being my faith for many years I asked myself to try and get a reason of why nature had made and placed in a person's head so much fine machinery just to make a little ear-wax. If nothing is made in vain, what is that bitter stuff made for? It is always there, and more being made all the time. I have read many authors or say so's about ear-wax, and about the best the wise or the unwise have said is that it would keep bugs and other insects out of our heads. I thought if that was all that it was made for nature had done a great deal to shoo off the bugs. The idea that it was made bitter and bad to eat just to make bugs sick was weak philosophy, if nature never did any useless work or made anything in vain. At this time I saw the doors all open and a good chance for the loaded mind to unload and give us other uses for ear-wax than bug food, and to lubricate the auditory nerves with dry wax. At this time of my desire to know some positive use or object that nature had in forming so much fine machinery and no use for its products when made, but to pull out of the head with a hairpin, I reasoned about so, that this dry hard wax was once in the gaseous or fluid state.

A SUCCESSFUL EXPERIMENT.

When I had about concluded to sit down with the common herd of doctors and say that wax was wax, a fat boy of two summers was reported to me to be dying with croup. I began to think more about the dry wax that is always found in cases of croup, sore throat, tonsilitis, pneumonia, and all diseases of the lungs, nose and head. On examination I found the ear-wax dried up. So I put a few drops of glycerine, and after a minute's time a few drops of warm water in the child's head, and kept a wet rag corked into its ear frequently for twelve hours, and gave it Osteopathic treatment, at the end of which time all signs of croup had disappeared. I used the glycerine to soften the wax, which combining with water formed a harmless soap better qualified for washing the ear, and retaining the wax in solution than anything I have tried, for it is my opinion that the ear wax should be kept in a fluid state. When in that state the absorbent can more readily take it up and use it in the economy of life in this condition. The same day two ladies came to my house, sore in lungs, necks tied up, sore throats, fever and headache. As an experiment, in addition to Osteopathic treatment, I put a few drops of glycerine in their ears, followed with water to wet and soften the wax which was dry and hard, to get it back to a fluid state. Both got better of their sore lungs and throats in a short time, and in twenty-four hours they were about well, and lungs coughing out phlegm, easily. From this I think that the cause of croup is simply the result of abnormality of the cerumen system.

A QUESTION FOR AGES.

As a question of the uses of ear-wax has been before man for ages without an answer being given that passes the line of conjecture, I think there could be no reason why a few looks through the field glass of inquiry should not be given in a limited way on that great plane of fertility, for the minds of our most profound thinkers. As far as the writer can learn from reading and other methods of inquiry, the power and use of ear-wax has never been known, looked on, or thought of as one of life's agents for good or bad health. One asks this question: "Why are you talking about ear-wax, the filthy stuff?" In answer I asked, "What do you know about ear-wax?" The answer, "I don't know or care anything about the dirty stuff."

THE POSITION.

As my spleen is my organ of mirth, I let it bounce against my side a few times at such ignorance and gave the wax subject more study than ever—I began to read all the books I could find on Anatomy, Physiology, and Histology to get some knowledge of the machinery that the wise architect of that greatest of all temples had made to generate wax. At this time a conviction came to me to be sure of its uses before I gave an opinion. I find the center of nerve supply of the ears located at the base of the brain and side of the head, in front of the cerebellum, just below and near the center of the brain, a little above the foramen magnum, close to and behind the carotid arteries, deep and superficial, just above the entry of the spinal cord to the brain. Thus it is situated directly in communication with all nerves to and from the brain to every part of the body. Another question, and another came only to come and go without an answer—such as how and where is this wax made? Of what use is it? Why so awful bitter? Has it any living principle above dry earth? Is it produced in the brain, lymphatics, fascia, heart, lungs, nerves or where? How much of it would kill a man? Would it kill at all? What is it made for? Is it used by nerves as food, or used by lungs, heart, or any organ as an active principle in the magnetic or electric forces? So far all authors are silent even to offer a speculative opinion about how it is made and its uses. So far we get nothing from the ancient or modern writers, as to its uses or anything that would cause a man to think that the Creator had any great design, when he made so wisely constructed and so much machinery and gave it such prominent place in the center of the brain. By this time the reader begins to mentally ask what does this wax evangelist know about the wax and its uses? The writer wishes to observe and respect all nature and never be too hasty. To carefully explore all, and never leave until he finds the cause and use that nature's hand has placed in its works, never overlooking small packages as they often contain precious gems. I am sure no man of brilliant mind can pass this milepost and not hitch his team and do some precious loading. At this point my pen will give notice to all anatomists, histologists, chemists and physiologists that I will give "no sleep nor slumber to their eyes," until I hear from them an answer, yes or no to these questions: For what purpose did God make ear-wax? Is it food or refuse? If food, what is nourished by it? and how do you know your position is true and undebatable?

MEANING OF LIFE.

Life means existence; existence means subsistence; subsistence means something to subsist on, and of the degree of refinement to suit the being or principle whose function is to do the skilled work which is found marked on the tressle-board of the wisest of all builders, whose work is absolutely correct in form and action, and beautiful to behold. It calls out the admiration of man and God himself, who did say of man, "Not only good, but very good."

SOME QUESTIONS ASKED.

I consider ear-wax one of the most important questions before the minds of our physiologists. The first and only knowledge of which substance begins with the observer's eye when he beholds the dry wax as it is excreted and dropped into the cavities of the ears. A question arises—and stands without an answer—is this substance which is commonly called ear-wax, technically called cerumen, is it dead or is it alive while in this form and visible? If dead, why, and how did it lose its life? Why has it not been consumed if once a living substance? When alive, is it in the gaseous or fluid state? and when alive, and consumed as nutriment by the system what does it nourish? is the question for the philosopher's attention, not superficial, but his deepest thought? Why is it deposited in the center of the brain if not to impart its vital principle to all nerves interested in life and nutrition—both physical and spiritual. Its location, itself, would indicate its importance. Another thought is that no better place could be selected to establish and locate a universal supply office for the laborers of all parts of the whole superstructure. Another question arises: When we examine a person paralyzed on one side, why do we find this bread of life in such great quantities on the table and not consumed? Has not one-half of the brain and the nerves of that whole side, limbs and all, lost their power of digestion? Is hemiplegia a dyspepsia of the nerves of nutriment of the brain and organs of that side? If so we have some foundation on which to build an answer why this wax is not consumed and is dried up in the ears of the parylytic. The answer would be that nutrition is suspended.

CONDITIONS IN CERTAIN DISEASES, CAUSED BY COLDS.

Let us take croup, diphtheria, scarlet fever, la grippe, and all classes of colds—on to pneumonia. They present about the same symptoms, differing more in degrees of severity than of place. All affect the tonsils, nostrils, membraneous air-passages, and lungs about the same way. Croup exceeds by contracting the trachea enough to impede the passing of air to the lungs; diphtheria has more swelling of the tonsils, throat and glands of the neck, but all depend upon the same blood and nerve supply, or a general law of blood beginning with arteries to and from veins, lymphatics, glands and ducts to supply and take away all fluids that are of no farther use to the vital and material support. As all authors have agreed that the brain furnishes the propelling forces to the nerves, it would be proper to inquire how the brain is nourished. If so, we will begin and say the great cerebral system of arteries supply the brain of which it gives quality of all fluids and electric and magnetic forces, which must be generated in the brain. Then a question arises, if the heart, lungs, liver, pancreas, lymphatics, kidneys and all parts of the body depend upon the brain for power, what do they give in return? If they give back anything it must be of the kind of the organ from whence it comes; thus a kidney cannot give liver nor spleen. Each must help to keep up the universal harmony by furnishing its mite of its own kind. Suppose lung fever is the effect of lack of renal salts, where would be a better place to dispatch from to renal organs than the ears to reach the brain and touch the nerve that connects with the sympathetic ganglion.

CERUMEN IN FLUID STATE.

Suppose we take the cerumen in its fluid state, by the secretions to the lungs from the ears and see the action of air and other substances on it, and it on them. We may safely look for a general action of some kind. If it be magnetic food, we will see the magnetic power shown in the lungs, and through the whole system, vitalizing all organs and functions of life. Thus the lymphatics will move to wash out impurities, and the nutritive nerves will rebuild lost energy. As but little is known or said of how or where the cerumen is formed, we will guess it is formed under the skin in the glands of the fascia and conveyed to the ears by the secretory ducts. Its place and how it is manufactured is not the question of the greatest importance, but its uses in disease and health.

WINTER KILLS BABIES.

The writer has much reason to believe he has found a reliable pointer for the cause of croup, diphtheria, and pneumonia; also a rational and easy cure that any mother can administer and save the babe from choking to death in her arms. Having witnessed croup in all its deadly work for fifty years, and seen the best skill of each year and generation fail to save, or even give relief, I lost all hope and grew to believe there was no help and the doctor was only one more witness to the scene of death and carnage found along the mysterious road that croup travels to slay the babes of the whole earth. Of later days we have new and different names for the disease, but alas, it kills the babe just as it did before it was called diphtheria, la grippe and so on.

SOME ADVICE TO MOTHERS.

I write this more for the mothers than for the critics. We say to mothers, as you are not Osteopaths, you are perfectly safe in putting glycerine in a child's ears. It is made from oils and fats. I believe when the wax is not consumed it clogs up the excretories with dead matter, thus the irritation of the nerves of throat, neck, lungs and lymphatics which give cause for the swelling of the tonsils and glands of the neck. In this book can be found why I see wisdom in treating for croup from the nerve centers of the brain. So far the uses and importance of healthy ear-wax as a cure for disease has had no attention that I can find by any author on disease or physiology. I hope time and attention may lead us to a better knowledge of the cure of diphtheria, croup, scarlet fever and all diseases of the throat and lungs of children, and how to cure a greater per cent than has been up to this writing. My experience up to date with such diseases, when treated as indicated, has been very encouraging. Though it is but a short time since I began to treat by this method, it has proven good with the young and old.

As all authors so far seem silent even as to how or when the wax is formed, we must resort to much careful dissection to find the relation of the cerumen system to health. To intelligently acquaint the mother with this treatment who does not understand anatomy so as to give Osteopathic treatment for croup, diphtheria, and so on, I will say; take a soft wet cloth and wash the child's neck and rub gently down from ears to breast and shoulders; keep ears wet, often dropping in the glycerine. Use glycerine because it will mix with the water and dissolve the wax, while sweet oil and other oils will not do so.

A CASE IN POINT.

At 2 o'clock p. m. I called to see a babe having malignant croup in its worst form, and examined its ears to see condition of wax. I had noticed in consumptives that some cases had great quantities of dry wax in one or both ears, but to this time had not thought of such deposits being an evidence of lost or suspended action of the nerves that manufactured cerumen. In this case I found wax dry and very hard, with much swelling and hardness in region of ears, eustachian tubes and tonsils. I reasoned that the excretory duct had become clogged, and that by the wax being retained in ducts and glands an irritation of the nerves of the cervical lymphatics had caused contraction near head, and produced congestion of the lymphatics, of the pneumogastric, and cutting off nerves supply from lungs. Believing this to be very likely I concluded to act on the above line of reasoning and see if I could give some relief. I did not stop to debate why the wax was hard and dry, but how to soften the wax, was the question of interest to me then. So I proceeded. I reasoned that soap and water would be the best treatment to clean the ears, and soften the wax. At this point to select the best make of soap in the ears was to be desired, so I took pure glycerine and water, dropped in a few drops and took a small roll of cloth, made it wet in warm water and pushed it in ears to keep them wet. In a few minutes I wet and inserted a soft cloth cork in the child's ears. I twisted the corks around in the ears, each time to mix the water and the wax to a softened condition, for to keep the wax wet was the object. In a few minutes I got the wax wet and the child coughed up phlegm easily, and when the dreaded hour, ten o'clock at night came, all danger had passed.

CONNECTION OF BRAIN AND OTHER NERVES IN DIGESTION.

If digestion is the effect of organs, fluids and forces, then the student of nature's law must be governed by well known truths, such as the location of the brain, connection of the nerves to other organs, bringing all parts interested in digestion in mental view. Thus you have a chance to know if one organ has an assisting relation to any other organ or system or if its products are of general or of special use. A few questions at this point of inquiry would be in place. Does the brain give assistance in digestion, and why may we reasonably suppose so, when digestion does its work normally and has a full, rich supply of blood? Yet disease enters the system, and begins its work with general weakness, swelling, wastings, and pain with some, or all the glands congested and sore, and a plenty of rich blood all the time. Then are we justified to go to the brain and examine the electric and magnetic batteries? We know such forces exist but as their location in the brain is not known farther than the fact of their existence, we do not know how they are fed, nor from where, so we are fully warranted in seeking a use for both powers—magnetic and electric. One says the power of electricity belongs more to the motor nerves and the magnetic to the nutrient system; if not they are happily blended and give the results. Without such forces life and motion could not be sustained. As it is not my object to write a treatise on general physiology, I will turn at once to the subject of the relation of life and health as affected by the abnormal supply and action of ear-wax.[3]

UNAIDED INVESTIGATION.

As our investigations are without the assistance of ancient or modern writers we will have to reason that man is a machine of form and power, forming its own parts and generating its own powers as it has use for them. At this time we begin to reason thus, that all powers are invisible and we see effect only. We know such forces to be abundant in nature, and life is sustained by them. To find the substances in the body that causes them to act and how to act, has been the object of my journey as an explorer. If they give us health when normal action prevails and disease only when abnormal, then we are admonished to form a more intimate acquaintance with the qualities, and with all the products, when formed in this great laboratory which compounds and qualifies each substance to fill its mission of force, construction, purity and action.

CHAPTER V.

DISEASES OF THE CHEST.

Where Confined—Consumption—Can Consumption Be Cured—
Consumption Described—No Time for Surrender—Cerebral Spinal
Fluid—How to Destroy Deadly Bombs of Decay—Battle of Blood for
Life—Militis Tuberculosis—Conversion of Bodies Into Gas—
Forming a Tubercle—Breeding Contagion—The Seeds of Disease—
Generating Fever—Whooping Cough—Clouds and Lungs Are Much
Alike—The Wisdom of Nature—Water Formed in Lungs—The Law
of Fives—Feeble Action of Heart—The Heart—From Neck to
Heart—Dyspepsia or Imperfect Digestion.

WHERE CONFINED.

Diseases of the chest are generally confined to heart, lungs, pleura, the pericardium, mediastium, blood vessels, with nerves and lymphatics. As we open the breast we behold the heart, a very large machine or engine, situated conveniently to throw blood to all parts of the body. To it we see hose or pipes that go to each organ, all muscles, the stomach, bowels, liver, spleen, kidneys, bladder and womb, all bones, fibers, ligaments, membranes, and its body, lungs and brain. When we follow this blood through its whole journey to feed the dependent parts, be they organ or muscle, we find just enough unloaded at each station to supply the demand as fast as consumed. Thus life is supplied at each stroke of the heart, which gives blood to keep digestion in full motion while other supplies of blood are being made and put in channels to carry to the heart, blood is freely given to keep those channels strong, clean and active. Thus much depends on the heart, and great care should be given to that study, because a healthy system depends almost wholly on a normal heart and lung. Thus to study well the frame work of the chest should be with the greatest care. Every joint of the neck and spine has much to do with a healthy heart and lung, because all vital fluids from crown to sacrum do or have passed through heart and lungs, and any slip of bone, strain or bruise will affect to some degree the usefulness of that fluid in its vitality, when appropriated in the place or organ it should sustain in a good healthy state. To the Osteopath, his first and last duty is to look well to a healthy blood and nerve supply. He should let his eye camp day and night on the spinal column; to know if the bones articulate truly in all facets and other bearings, and never rest day or night until he knows the spine is true and in line from atlas to sacrum, with all ribs known to be in perfect union with processes of spine. In reasoning for probable causes of diseases of chest, we are met with the fact that the heart and lungs are housed up, and out of reach of the hand and eye. We hear a cough, see blood and other substances after they pass out of the lungs; we learn of general and local pain and misery, feel heat and cold on skin, note abnormal breathing, but here we are at a stop, for want of facts. We know something is wrong, but cannot say what, until after death has done the work, then we open the chest and find tubercles, cancers, ulcers and abcesses. How came they there? is the unanswered question. The servant of that breast who failed to keep his room clean, is the one to find and punish.

CONSUMPTION.

I believe so much death by consumption will soon be with the things of the past, if the cases are taken early and handled by a skilled mind,—one trained for that responsible place. He or she must be taught this as a special branch. It is too deep for superficial knowledge or imperfect work. Life is in danger, and can be saved by skill, not by force and ignorance. He who sees only the dollar in the lung, is not the man to trust with your case.

It is such men as have the ability to think, and the skill to comprehend and execute the application of nature's unerring laws, that obtain the results required. We believe the day has come, and long before noon, the fear of consumption will greatly pass from the minds of people. We have long since known and proven that a cough is only an effect. If an effect then a wise man will set his mental dogs on the track, which is (effect) to hunt the skunk, (cause). He has all the evidence by the cough, location of pain, tenderness of spine, neck, and quality of the substances coughed up to locate the cause, and to know, when he has found it, how to remove the cause, and give relief; will grow more simple as he reasons and notes effect.

We do not think this result will be obtained every time by even an average mind, unless he has a special training for that purpose. He must not only know that the lungs are in the upper part of the chest close to the heart, liver and stomach, but he must know the relation all sustain to each other, that the blood must be abundantly supplied, support and nourish three sets of nerves, namely sensory, motor and nutrient; also voluntary and involuntary. If the supply should be diminished on the nutrient nerves, weakness would follow; reduce the supply from the motor and it will have the same effect. Motion becomes too feeble to carry blood to and from lungs normally, and the blood becomes diseased and congested, because it is not passed on to other parts with the force necessary for health of lungs.

At this time the nerves of sensation become irritated by pressure and lack of nutriment, and we cough, which is an effort of nature to unload the burden of oppression that congestion causes with sensory nerves. If this be effect, then we must suffer and die, or remove the cause, put out the fire and stop waste of life, without which all is lost. Nature will do its work of repairing in due time. Let us reason by comparison. If we dislocate a shoulder, fever and heat will follow. The same is true of all limbs and joints of the body. If any obstructing blood or other fluid should be deposited in quantities great enough to stop other fluids from passing on their way, Nature will fire up its engine to remove such deposits by converting fluids into gas. As heat and motion have much to do as remedies, we may expect fever and pain until nature's furnace produces heat, forms and converts its fluids into gas and other deposits, and passes them through the excretories to space, and allows the body to work normally again.

HOW CONSUMPTION USUALLY BEGINS.

We believe consumption causes the death of thousands annually who might be saved. We must not let stupidity veil our reason, and we are to blame if we let so many run into "Consumption" from a simple hard cough. The remedy is natural, and we believe from results already obtained 75 per cent can be cured if taken in time. What we generally call "Consumption" begins with a cough, chilly sensations, and lasts a day or two. Sometimes fever accompanies with cough, either high or low. The cold generally relaxes in a few days, lungs get "loose," and much is raised and continues for a period, but the cough appears again and again with all changes of weather, and lasts longer each time, until it becomes permanent, then it is called "Consumption," because of this continuance. Medicines are administered freely and often, but the lungs grow worse, cough more continued and much harder, till finally blood begins to come from lungs with wasting of strength. Change of climate is suggested and taken, but with no change for the better; another and another travels to death on the same line. Then the doctor in council reports "hereditary consumption" and with his decision all are satisfied, and each member of the family feels that a cold and cough means a coffin, because the doctor says the family has "hereditary consumption." This shade tree has given comfort and contentment to the doctors of the whole past.

CAN CONSUMPTION BE CURED?

If you have a tiresome and weakening cough at the close of the winter, and wish to be cured, we would advise you to begin Osteopathic treatment at once, so the lungs can heal and harden against next winter's attack.

This is the first I have written on "Consumption" because I wanted to test my conclusions by long and careful observations on cases that I have taken and successfully treated. I kept the results from public print until I could obtain positive proof that "Consumption" could be cured. So far the discovered causes give me little doubt, and the cures are a certainty in very many cases. An early beginning is one of the great considerations in incipient consumption.

CONSUMPTION DESCRIBED.

For fear you do not understand what I mean by "Consumption" I will write on a descriptive line quite pointedly. I will give start and progress to fully developed consumption. We often meet with cases of permanent cough, with expectorations of long duration, dating back two, five, ten, even thirty years, to the time they had measles. The severity of the cough and strain had congested even the lung substances, and a chronic inflammation was the result. If we analyze the sputa we find fibrin and even lung muscle. Does all this array of dangerous symptoms cause an Osteopath to give up in despair? It should not, on the other hand he should go deeper on the hunt of cause. He may find trouble in nerve fiber of pneumogastric nerve, atlas or hyoid, vertebra, rib, or clavicle, may be by pressing on some nerve that supplies mucous membrane of air cells or passages. A cut foot will often produce lockjaw, why not a pressure on some center branch or nerve fiber cause some division—nerve of the lungs that governs venous circulation which would contract and hold blood indefinitely as an irritant, equal to cause, perpetual coughing?

NO TIME FOR SURRENDER.

This is not the time for the brainy Osteopath to run up the white flag of defeat and surrender. Open the doors of your purest reason, put on the belt of energy and unload the sinking vessel of life. Throw overboard all dead weights from fascia and wake up the forces of the excretories. Let the nerves all show their powers to throw out every weight that would sink or reduce the vital energies of nature. Give them a chance to work, give them the full nourishment and the victory will be on the side of the intelligent engineer. Never surrender but die in the last ditch.

Let us enter the field of active exploration and note the causes that would lead us to conclude we have the cause that produces "consumption" as it has ever been called.

Begin at the brain, go down the ladder of observation, stop and whet your knives of mental steel sharp, get your nerves quiet by the opium of patience. Begin with the atlas, follow with the search-light of quickened reason, comb back your hair of mental strength, and never leave that bone till you have learned how many nerves pass through and around that wisely formed first part of the neck. Remember it was planned and builded by the mind and hand of the infinite. See what nerve fibers passes through and on to the base center, and each minute cell, fascia, gland and blood vessel of the lungs. Do you not know that each nerve fiber to its place is king and lord of all?

CEREBRAL SPINAL FLUID.

I think consumption begins by closing the channels of cerebro-spinal fluid in neck, which fluid stands as one of, if not the most highly refined elements in animal bodies. Its fineness would indicate that it is a substance that must be delivered in full supply continually to keep health normal; if so, we will for experimental reasons look at the neck ligated, as found in measles, croup, colds and eruptive fevers. Supply is stopped from passing below atlas for three days. During such diseases fever runs high at this time and dries up the albumen, giving cause for tubercles to begin, as fever has dried out the water and left the albumen in small deposits in the lungs, liver, kidneys and bowels. If this view of the great uses of brain fluid is true as cause of glandular growths and other dead deposits; have we not a cause for militis tuberculosis? Have we not encouragement to prosecute with interest, in the hope of an answer to the question, "What is tuberculosis?" Our writers are just as much at sea to-day as a thousand years ago. I will give the reader some of the reasons why I think the mischief was started while fluid was cut off by congestion of neck. How can the fluid be cut off at neck is a very natural question. By the crudest method of reasoning we would conclude that from the form of the neck, many objects are indicated, and the material of which it is composed would give reason to turn all its powers of thought, to ask why it is so formed, as to twist, bend, straighten, stiffen and relax at will, to suit so many purposes? A very tough skin—a sheathe—surrounds the neck with blood vessels, nerves, muscles, bones, ligaments, fascia, glands great and small, throat and trachea. In bones we find a great canal for spinal cord. It is well and powerfully protected by a strong wall of bone, so no outer pressure can obstruct the flow of passing fluids, to keep vitality supplied by brain forces, but with all the guards given to protect the cord, we find that it can be overcome by impact fluids to such degree as to stop blood and other fluids from supplying lungs and all below.

The fluid we speak of comes from the skull, and when in process of formation must not be disturbed until it has passed through all chances of being injured by force, air or light. Thus the great need of walls to hold the enemy outside the safety line. Such truths surely should attract our attention when we explore for causes. We can analyze material bodies but we have to stop at the life line for more knowledge. Our boats have been in port over 6000 years, waiting for knowledge about the whats and whys of life, until barnacles of ignorance have accumulated to such thickness that the conchologist has called that cake of shells "allopathy" which weighed anchor and turned to the great sea of human credulity to expound, with nothing but conjectures to offer. He toots his fog-horn in all lands and on all seas, and says, "age before reason." Thus one generation blindly follows another.

HOW TO DESTROY DEADLY BOMBS OF DECAY.

I think by this time the reader has gotten his mind in line with his exploring needle of thought to get some light or knowledge of why a growth and how a body that has never failed for few or many years, begins and continues to form and plant deadly bombs of decay in that once powerful engine of perfect health, to produce suicide. We see and know this to be the case in thousands of beings annually, and this same question is just as applicable to the herds of animals as to man. Thus we cry piteously for help, but no answer has come in past days; we go on and give place in lungs and other parts of the deadly tubercle. But one answer can be given in "Holy Writ" to suit these questions, "Cleanliness is next to Godliness." Turn the waters of life loose at the brain, remove all hindrances and the work will be done, and give us the eternal legacy, LONGEVITY.

BATTLE OF BLOOD FOR LIFE.

In America from the day of Washington and all centuries before his time, man has dreaded diseases of the lungs more universally than any other one disease. If we compare pulmonary diseases with other maladies we find more persons die of consumption, pneumonia, bronchitis and nervous coughs than from smallpox, typhus and bilious fever and all other fevers combined. Many diseases of contagious natures do not stay in city, town, country nor an army, but a short time; kills a few and disappears and may not return for many years. The same is the history of yellow fever, cholera and other epidemics. They slay their hundreds and stop as unceremoniously as they began. But when we think of diseases that begin to show their effects in tonsils, trachea and lining membranes of the air passages, we find we are in a boundless ocean; because we find all seasons of the year, which afford changes of weather: Wet, dry, windy, hot and cold, which mark 30° to 60° in twenty-four hours, chills the lungs and whole system, closes the excretory system against renovating equal to deposits, with all other chances to throw out dead matter and gases that destroy blood and life in proportion to the amount and time of abnormal retention.

It takes no great mind to know from past observation that a common cold often holds on and settles down to chronic inflammation of the lungs, and the patient dies of consumption, croup, diphtheria, tonsilitis, and as catarrhal trouble stays and begins to waste vitality by failing to oxygenize blood while in the lungs, diphtheria paves the way for the young and old to die of consumption. Dance halls, opera houses, churches, school houses, and all crowded assemblies never fail to inspect and deposit the seeds of consumption in weak lungs.

As one delves deeper and deeper into the machinery and exacting laws of life, he beholds works and workings of contented laborers of all parts of the one common whole—the great shafts and pillars of an engine working to the fullness of the meaning of perfection. He sees that great quarter-master the heart, pouring in and loading train after train and giving orders to the wagon-master to line his teams and march on quick time to all divisions, supply all companies, squads and sections with rations, clothing, ammunition, surgeons, splints and bandages, and put all the dead and wounded into the ambulances to be repaired or buried with military honors by Captain "VEIN," who fearlessly penetrates the densest bones, muscles and glands, with the living waters to quench the thirst of the blue corpuscles, who are worn out by doing fatigue duty in the great combat between life and death. He often has to run his trains on forced marches to get supplies to sustain his men of life when they have had to contend with long sieges of heat and cold. Of all officers of life, none have greater duties to perform than the quarter-master of blood supply, who borrows the force with which he runs his deliveries from the brain which give motion to all parts of active life.

MILITIS TUBERCULOSIS.

A tubercle is a separate body being enveloped.[4]

As all descriptions of a tubercle in books amount to about this, that the tubercle is an amount of fleshy substance which may be albumen, fibrin, or any other substance collected and deposited at one place in the human body, and covered with a film composed generally of fibrinous substances, and deposited in its spherical form, and separated from all similarly formed spheres by fascia. They may be very numerous, for many hundreds may occupy one cubic inch and yet one is distinct from all others. They seem to develop only where fascia is abundant; in the lungs, liver, bowels and skin. After formation they may exist and show nothing but roughened surfaces, and when the period of dissolution and the solvent powers of the chemical laboratory take possession to banish them from the system, it generally begins its labors at such time as some catarrhal disease is preying upon the human system. Nature seems to make its first effort for the purpose of disposing of such substances as have accumulated at the catarrhal period. At which time it brings forward all the solvent qualities and applies them with the assistance of the motor force to drive out through the bowels, lungs, porous and excretory system all irritable substances. Electricity is called in as the motor force to be used in expelling all unkindly substances. By this effort of nature, which is an increased action of the motor nerves, electricity is brought to the degree of heat usually called fever, which if better understood we would possibly find to be the necessary heat of the furnace of the body being used to convert dead substances into gas which can travel through the excretory system and be thrown from the body much easier than water, lymph, albumen or fibrin.

CONVERSION OF BODIES INTO GAS.

During this process of gas burning, a very high temperature is obtained by the increased action of the arterial system through the motor nerves, permeating those tubercles and causing an inflammation of them by the gaseous disturbance so produced; another effort of nature to convert those tubercles into gas and relieve the body of their presence and irritable occupancy.

As an illustration we will ask the reader if it would be reasonable to expect to pass a common towel through a pipe stem. Nevertheless nature can easily do it. Confine the towel in a cylinder and apply fire, which in time will convert the towel into gas or smoke, and enable it to pass through the stem. Is it not just as reasonable to suppose those high temperatures of the body are nature's furnaces, making fires out of those dead bodies, while passing them through the skin in order to get rid of these great and small towels which are packed all through the human fascia, and can only be passed from the body in a gaseous form; the gas generated by heat.

The blackened eye of the pugilist soon fires up its furnaces and proceeds to generate gas from the dead blood that surrounds the eye. Though it may be considerable quantities under the skin, the blood soon disappears leaving the face and eye normal to all appearances. No pus has formed, nor deposit left, fever disappears, the eye is well. What better effort could nature offer than through its gas generating furnace. I will leave any other method for you to discover. I know of none that my reason can grasp.

FORMING A TUBERCLE.

When reason sees a white corpuscle in the fascia not taken up as a nutrient, it attaches itself to the fascia with all its uterine powers during the time of measles or other eruptive diseases, and soon takes form and is a vital and durable being whose name is tubercle; in form a sphere, and place of fœtal life is a cell in the fascia of life giving power to all forms of flesh. Thus all tubercles are unappropriated substances whom mother fascia has clothed and ordered in camp for treatment and repairs, and placed them on the list of enrolled pensioners, to draw on the treasury of the fascia, until death shall discharge them.

BREEDING CONTAGION.

The mothers of the human race give birth to children from puberty to sterility. She may give birth a dozen times, but nature finally calls a halt, and the whole system of life sustaining nerves of the womb which are in the fascia, with blood in great abundance to supply fœtal life, ceases to go farther with the processes of building beings. Vitality for that purpose stops, never to return. Nature has no longer a demand for her system to act as a constructing cause for other beings, of her kind, and she is free the remainder of her days.

A question arises. Are children all she can develop in her system and give birth to? No, she can go through other processes of breeding. In her fascia there is one seed, if vitalized will develop a being called measles. She never has but one confinement. That set of nerves that gave support and growth to measles died in the delivery of the child, and never can conceive and produce any more measles. Another seed lives in her fascia waiting to be vitalized by the male principle of smallpox, and when it is born it always kills the nerves that gave it life and form. And the person never can have but one such child or being during life.

Still another seed awaits the coming of the commissary to nourish while it consumes that vitality in the fascia of the glands to develop the portly child we call mumps. Both male and female conceive and give birth to such beings, then tear up the tracks and roads behind them, by killing the demand for such drink.

I want to draw the mind of the reader to the fact that no being can be formed without material. A place in which to be developed, and all forces necessary to do the needed work. And as all excrescences and abnormal growths, diseases and conditions, must have the friendly assistance of the fascia before development; the fascia is the place to look for cause of disease and the place to consult and begin the action of remedies in all diseases, even though it be the birth of a child.

THE SEEDS OF DISEASE.

We can arrive at truth only by the powerful rules of reason, so the philosopher has shouted from the house tops of all ages. He adjusts his many supposable causes, adds to and subtracts until he arrives at a conclusion based upon the facts of his observations. Knowing the principles that exist in substances and seeds, by which when associated with proper conditions that powerful engine known as animal life gives the truth with fact and motion as its voucher. We reason, if corn be planted in moist and warm earth, that action and growth will present the form of a living stalk of corn, which has existed in embryo, and still continues its vital actions as long as the proper conditions prevail, i. e., until the growth and development is completed. If you take a seed in your fingers, push it in the ground and cover it up, incubation, growth and development is expected in obedience to the law under which it serves. Thus we see to succeed we must deposit and cover up the seed in order that the laws of gestation may have an opportunity by which they get the results desired. As nature always presents itself to our minds as seeds deposited in soil and season to suit, and it is loyal to its own laws only, we are constrained by this method of reasoning to conclude that disease must have a soil in which to plant its seeds before gestation and development. It must have seasonable conditions, the rains of nourishment, also the necessary time required for such processes. All these laws must be fulfilled to the letter, otherwise a failure is absolute. As the great laboratory of nature is always at work in the human body, the chilling winds and poisonous breaths, with extremes of heat and cold at different seasons of the year by day and night, and the lungs and skin are continually secreting and excreting every minute, hour and day of our lives, is it not reasonable to suppose that we inhale many elements that are floating in the common winds that contain the seeds of some destructive element, to the harmony of fluids that are necessary to sustain the healthy animal forms.

GENERATING FEVER.

Suppose it should start the yeast, or kind of substance that lives greatly upon lime. If this yeast in its action and thirst for food to suit its life and appetite should call in from the earth, water and atmosphere for its daily food lime substances only, and by its power destroy all other principles taken as nourishment, is it not reasonable to suppose it would deposit such elements in over powering quantities in the fascia of the mucous membrane of the lungs in such quantities, as to overcome the renovating powers of the lungs and excretory system, by its paralyzing quantities of diseased fluids, all through the universal fascia of animal life. This deposit acts as an irritant to the sensory nerves to such an extent that the electricity of the motor nerves is forced to take charge of, and run the machinery of the human body, with such velocity as to raise the temperature of the body, by putting the electricity above the normal action of animal life, and thereby generate that temperature known as fever?

The two extremes, heat and cold, may be the causes of retention and detention. One is detained by the contraction of cold until the blood and other fluids die by asphyxia. The warm temperature produces relaxation of the nerves, blood, and all other vessels of the fascia, during which time the arteries are injecting too great quantities of fluids to be renovated by the excretory systems. Thus you have a cause for decomposition of the blood and other substances, to be conveyed to the lungs for purification and renewal. You have a logical foundation and a cause for all diseases, catarrhal, climatic, contagions, infections, and epidemics. The fascia proves itself to be the probable matrix of life and death. Beginning with the mucous membrane penetrating all parts to supply and renovate the fluids of life, and nourishing all the nerves of nutrition and assimilation. When harmonious in normal action, health is good; when perverted, disease is destructive unto death.

WHOOPING COUGH.

I have perused all the authority obtainable, advised with and counciled for information in reference to the cause of whooping cough until I am constrained to think, whether I say so or not, that I have had many additions of words during the conversation, and to use a homely phrase, less sense than I started out with. My tongue is tired, my brain exhausted, my hopes disappointed and my mind disgusted, that after so much effort to obtain some positive knowledge of the disease in question, which is whooping cough, that I have received nothing that would give me any light whatever pertaining to the subject. It winds up thus, that it may be a germ that irritates the pneumogastric nerve. I go off as blank and empty as the fish lakes on the moon. I supposed writers would say something in reference to the irritating influence of this disease on the nerves and muscles that would contract or convulsively shorten the muscles that attach at the one end to the os hyoid, and at the other end at various points along the neck, and force the hyoid back against the pneumogastric nerve, hypoglossal, cervical, or some other nerve that would be irritated by such pressure on nerves by the os hyoid, when pulled back and held against such nerves. The above picture will give the reader some idea why I became so thoroughly disgusted with the heaps of compiled trash. I say trash because there was not a single truth, great or small, to guide me in search of the desired knowledge. And at this point I will say on my first exploration I found all of the nerves and muscles that attach to the os hyoid at any point contracted, shortened and pulling the hyoid back to and pressing against the pneumogastric nerve, and all the nerves in that vicinity. Also each and every muscle was in a hard and contracted condition in the region of this portion of the trachea, and extended up and into the back part of the tongue. Then I satisfied myself that this irritable condition of the muscles was possibly the cause of the spasms of the trachea during the convulsive cough. I proceeded at once with my hand guided by my judgment to suspend or stop for awhile the action of the nerves of sensation that go with and control the muscles of the machinery which conducts air to and from the lungs. That my first effort while acting upon this philosophy was a complete relaxation of all muscles and fibers of that part of the neck, and when they relaxed their hold upon the respiratory machinery the breathing became normal. I have been asked what bone I would pull when treating whooping cough? My answer would be, the bones that held by attachment the muscles of the hyoid system in such irritable condition that begin with the atlas and terminate with the sacrum. To him who has been a willing student of the American School of Osteopathy the successful management of whooping cough should be absolute, reliable and successful in all cases, when taken for treatment in anything like, a reasonable time.

CLOUDS AND LUNGS ARE MUCH ALIKE.

One is always the same in form and stays in the body of animals, while the clouds, the lungs of the sky, are never the same in form. They are sometimes very dense and separated from all others. Such are more furious in display. Then we see the softer clouds which cover all visible space above; they too give us rain but in a more quiet way and are more extended in space; they shade the sun, and form water by uniting oxygen and hydrogen, and supply vegetation and all demands for water. Now we see and know the uses for the clouds or lungs of the sky, and we are led to hunt and locate the water forming clouds of the animal beings. As we behold above us the forming clouds we see great activity, with darkness and attending shadows, without such shadows or darkness no rain can form.

The lung of man, too, is in the shade, and surely like the clouds have much to do with the air which contains both gases, which compose water and other elements of life. With my power of reasoning, if the lungs do not generate water and supply the human system through the secretions to sustain life, and keep the body clean and healthy by the excretories, I am at a loss to know why so much wind is taken into the body just to blow out. One would say we live by the wind, and to cut it off we die. At this point I will ask the question, Where and how do fishes get their wind? If they can live on oxygen and hydrogen when united in the form of water, is not this the strongest conclusion we can come to that the lungs generate water of a purer quality than is found in the running brooks or ocean?

Is it not reasonable to suppose that in the lungs can be found the fountain from which water is conveyed to the lymphatics and other parts of the body, to mix with the blood and keep it in proper condition while in construction and processes of renovation? Then if this be true, have we not established and located the fountain head and supply of the nutrient waters of life? If so are we not justified in going to that fountain for water to extinguish a fire that is consuming the body, which we call fever? This heat never appears until the water supplying the lymphatics is very much exhausted, previous to this exhibition of heat; which the chemist would conclude was the result of the action of phosphorous uniting with oxygen without hydrogen.

We as philosophical machinists, to extinguish this fire by every method of reason, would be forced to go to the lungs, and place them in a condition that they can generate water at once and supply the excretory ducts, which will at the first pulsation of the heart throw water upon the consuming fire, and extinguish it by uniting oxygen with hydrogen, and cover the burning building with water by disabling the power of phosphorous and oxygen from uniting and keeping up the flames of destruction.

THE WISDOM OF NATURE.

For all my life previous to the day I spoke out with my conclusions of the wisdom of nature as a very wise and careful mechanic, I had been told that "God" was wise to a finish,—from my birth until I was thirty-five years old,—when I saw that all work done by that law of power and wisdom was absolutely perfect in all its requirements. In vegetable life no power of human can detect a flaw or even suggest an additional leaf, limb or fruit. I had made a long study of minerology in which I found each stone or mettle was in a division of life that was its own, and no other stone could appear dressed in its garb, from the black silurian to the purely transparent crystal. I saw that a diamond could not be a ruby, neither could it be an oak, a goose nor a goat. With all the teaching which had given God credit for his perfect construction, wisdom and ability in all nature, I reasoned that in parching seasons that the sun's fires were put out, and a feverish earth cooled by the falling dews of the clouds. I asked of my own reason if there was not a cloud of water in the human body that could be caused to drop its dews, put out the fires of fever, and save the forests of life that were being burned every fall season.

WATER FORMED IN LUNGS.

I reasoned that water was made by the union of two gases, hydrogen and oxygen,—then a question arose, Is it not fully in line with reason that union of the two gases can and does occur in the lungs and form water, that is taken up by the secretions carried to the lymphatics, and by them to all of the system and stored away for use? Thus I reasoned, and proceeded to seek nerve centers to cause the lymphatics to discharge this water on such places and in quantities sufficient to reduce the heat called fever. I succeeded, fevers vanished as with a magic touch, and left the persons, both old and young, in their normal temperatures without any difference as to kinds of fever to the complete list.

Our lungs are surely the half-way place between life and death. We are told by chemistry that two gases make water for the uses of the body. Is it not true that nature makes water in great quantities often for special cases or conditions, for relief purposes, such as in asiatic cholera, cholera morbus, chills and fever; when the contents of stomach, bowels and skin run off many gallons of water, running through sheet and mattress and on floor, not from kidneys but skin. Is it not plain to the man of reason that the two gases, oxygen and hydrogen, do unite in the lungs, form water and give supply to this great river of water that washes life out in but a few hours in cases of cholera and other diseases. The person is very cold at such times, breath and lung far below the normal, and fully enough to condense gases to water.

THE LAW OF FIVES.

Lungs have five lobes, three on right lung, and two on left. Liver has five lobes, three on right lobe, and two on left lobe. Nerves have five qualities, nutrition, sensation, motion, voluntary and involuntary. Nerves have five senses, seeing, hearing, feeling, smelling and tasting. Since all principles differ in qualities or kinds of service, would it be amiss for us to inquire a little farther why the lungs and liver are provided with five divisions each, if not to do five kinds of work, and different from all other kinds in many ways?

FEEBLE ACTION OF HEART.

I want to draw your attention to the facts that there is no method known by which electricity or magnetic forces can be weighed. When we find the nerves that connect the heart and lungs to brain limited by pressure from twist or slip of neck, do we not see cause for croup? How would we reason to convey electricity without a connected wire? Not at all, we would know no electric force could reach to any point unless a continued connection was made. Now to the point; suppose the vagus nerve should be oppressed to a condition to cut off part of the electricity, would we be surprised if the heart should be feeble in action. I think much of the diseases of the *"heart"* are not of the organ but from a feeble supply of electricity that is cut off in medulla or heart nerves, between heart and brain. Why singing and roaring of ears in heart diseases, if there is no waste of pectoral electricity?

THE HEART.

With the knife of reason in hand and the microscope of mind of the greatest known power properly adjusted, we cut and lay open the breast of man. Here we dwell indefinitely. This is the engine of life, the self-propelling machine which has constructed all that is necessary to its own convenience and comfort. It has brought and deposited its own nourishment in the coronary arteries, whose duty is to construct and enlarge the heart from time to time as its demands increase. We see its main trunk of supply placed lengthways with the spinal column for the purpose of constructing a manufactory of nutriment. We pass from the heart upward about one foot, here we find it has constructed a battery of force and sensation, and contains all power necessary to carry on construction to the completed man.

In that brain or battery is found all the motor and sensory elements of life, with nerves to transmit all nerve powers and principles found in the human body. There is not a known atom in the whole human make-up that has not been propelled by the heart through the channels by which it has provided for such purpose. Every muscle, bone, hair, and all other parts without an exception have traveled through this system of arteries to their separate destinations. All are indebted to the heart for their material size, and all qualities of motion and life sustaining principles of the human body.

If the carotid artery should tire out and not be able to perform its duty the brain would tire out also, and cease to operate. Should the descending aorta come to a halt from any cause, all parts of the body depending upon that vessel would suffer a total loss of blood supply. Equally so with any other principal artery of limb or body, all mark a failure equal to the suspended supply. The parts and principles of the human body depending upon the heart are numerous beyond computation. Every expulsive stroke of the heart throws into line armed and equipped for duty thousands and millions of operators, whose duties are to inspect, repair injuries and construct anew if need be from the crown of the head to the sole of the foot. With the best eye of reason we see but dimly into the breast of man which contains the heart, the wonder of man and the secret of life.

I have given these bulky descriptions of the forest and ocean to prepare the mind of man to begin the inspection of the machinery that has constructed the body of which he is the indweller. If we cannot swallow all, we can taste.

FROM NECK TO HEART.

The hearts of all animals should call the most careful attention of the student of nature. He finds in it the first act of life; from it go all parts or by it all parts of the body are made, and the student of nature soon learns that at the heart he finds the first evidence of the power of life to continue and give useful shape to matter. Its first work is to complete itself in material form with necessary chambers to hold blood and with tubes to convey to all places of need. He sees vessels leaving the heart to form brain, lungs, liver, trunk and limbs, and with each and all he can see the nerves of motion, sensation, nutrition, the voluntary and involuntary—all working in perfect harmony and content to do their part in the economy of life. Without that union in action a confusion will show in form of abnormality which is known as disease. On its work all nerves do depend for force and strength to build and renovate the body in all its bones, muscles and nerves—thus all channels to and from the heart must be cleared from all hindrance. No nerve can do its part unless it be well nourished. If not it will fail to execute its part for want of power—for by it all blood must move. These nerves are found in plexuses in all parts of the body; they are abundant in the skin, fascia, muscle, lymphatics and all organs great and small. The Osteopath must know or learn that no infringement can be tolerated in any part. Nature's demands are surely absolute, and require that the last farthing shall be paid in full. Now for a start—we will explore the neck; here we have the great and small occipital and the cervical group all receiving from the brain and feeding parts below. Thus we must stop at the neck and read the lessons that can be found there, and learn them well; or we will find that we will not be able to meet diseases only to be defeated. We must have the fight during the four seasons of the year. In the cold seasons we will find lung and other diseases—croup, pneumonia, diphtheria, sore throat. All these do their mischief through the nerves of the neck.

Where is or who is the great thinker who knows and can tell all of the duties and actions of the nerves of the neck, or what nerve failed and slept while a tubercle was formed in the lungs? Which nerve slept while fat is heaped up in useless piles in the body? Let us wake up! Consumption does not come without a cause. What plexus is overcome and allows the lungs to waste away? To what ganglion of the spine would the finger of reason point, and say, "that is the cause of *phthisis pulmonalis*?" In our search we find a division of nerves run from the brain through the regions of the neck, and find a point at which a branch leaves a greater nerve on a line that leads to the lungs. We will likely find a ganglion at which place all or much of one or both lungs are supplied. Then we, by reason, would see that freedom of action cannot be. If some substance should intrude by pressure on any nerve in that region, we must judge by conditions if that pressure has cut off nutrition equal to feeble condition of the lungs.

DYSPEPSIA OR IMPERFECT DIGESTION.

In our physiologies we read much about digestion. We will start in where they stop. They bring us to the lungs with chyle fresh as made and placed in thoracic duct, previous to flowing into the heart to be transferred to lungs to be purified, charged with oxygen and otherwise qualified, and sent off for duty, through the arteries great and small, to the various parts of the system. But there is nothing said of the time when all blood is gas (if ever) before it is taken up by the secretions, after refinement, and driven to the lungs to be mixed with the old blood from the venous system. A few questions about the blood seem to hang around my mental crib for food. Reason says we cannot use blood before it has all passed through the gaseous stage of refinement, which reduces all material to the lowest forms of atoms, before constructing any material body. I think it safe to assume that all muscles and bones of our body have been in the gas state while in the process of preparing substances for blood. A world of questions arise at this point.

QUESTIONS OF GAS.

The first is, Where and how is food made into gas while in the body? If you will listen to a dyspeptic after eating you will wonder where he gets all the wind that he rifts from his stomach, and continues for one or two hours after each meal. That gas is generated in the stomach and intestines, and we are led to believe so because we know of no other place in which it can be made and thrown into the stomach by any tubes or other methods of entry. Thus by the evidence so far the stomach and bowels are the one place in which this gas is generated. Now comes question two: As I have spoken of the stomach that generates and ejects great quantities of gas for a longer or shorter time after meals, this class of people have always been called dyspeptics. Another class of the same race of beings stand side by side with him, without this gas generating. He, too, eats and drinks of the same kind of food, without any of the manifestations that have been described in the first class. Why does one stomach blow off gas continually, while the other does not? is a very deep, serious and interesting question. As number two throws off no gas from the stomach after eating, is this conclusive evidence that his stomach generates no gas? Or does his stomach and bowels form gas just as fast as No. 1? and the secretions of the stomach and bowels take up and retain the nutritious matter and pass the remainder of the gas by way of the excretory ducts through the skin? If the excretory ducts take up and carry this gas out of the body by way of the skin, and he is a healthy man, why not account for No. one's stomach ejecting this gas by way of the mouth, because of the fact that the secretions of the stomach are either clogged up or inactive, for want of vital motion of the nerve terminals of the stomach. Another question in connection with this subject: Why is the man whose stomach belches forth gas in such abundance also suffering with cold feet, hands and all over the body, while No. 2 is quite warm and comfortable, with a glow of warmth passing from his body all the time? With these hints I will ask the question: What is digestion?

CHAPTER VI.

THE LYMPHATICS.

Importance of the Subject—Demands of Nature on the Lymphatics—
Dunglinson's Definition—Dangers of Dead Substances—Lymph
Continued—Solvent in Nature—Where Are the Lymphatics
Situated?—The Fat and Lean.

IMPORTANCE OF THE SUBJECT.

Possibly less is known of the lymphatics than any other division of
the life-sustaining machinery of man. Thus ignorance of that division
is equal to a total blank with the operator. Finer nerves dwell with
the lymphatics than even with the eye. The eye is an organized
effect, the lymphatics the cause; in them the spirit of life more
abundantly dwells. No atom can leave the lymphatics in an
imperfect state and get a union with any part of the body. There the
atom obtains form and knowledge of how and what to do. The
lymphatics consume more of the finer fluids of the brain than the
whole viscera combined. By nature, coarser substances are necessary
to construct the organs that run the blast, and rough forging
divisions. The lymphatics form, finish, temper and send the bricks to
the builder with intelligence, that he may construct by adjusting all
according to nature's plans and specifications. Nature makes
machinery that can produce just what is necessary, and when united,
produces what the most capable minds could exact.

The lymphatics are closely and universally connected with the spinal
cord and all other nerves, long or short, universal or separate, and all
drink from the waters of the brain. By an action of the nerves of the
lymphatics, a union of qualities necessary to produce gall, sugar,
acids, alkalies, bone, muscle and softer parts, with the thought that
elements can be changed, suspended, collected and associated and
produce any chemical compound necessary to sustain animal life,
wash out, salt, sweeten and preserve the being from decay and death
by chemical, electric, atmospheric or climatic conditions. By this we
are admonished in all our treatment not to wound the lymphatics, as

they are undoubtedly the life giving centers and organs. Thus it behooves us to handle them with wisdom and tenderness, for by and from them a withered limb, organ or any division of the body receives what we call reconstruction, or is builded anew, and without this cautious procedure your patient had better save his life and money by passing you by as a failure, until you are by knowledge qualified to deal with the lymphatics.

DEMANDS OF NATURE ON THE LYMPHATICS.

Why not reason on the broad plain of known facts, and give the why he or she has complete prostration. When all systems are cut off from a chance to move and execute such duties as nature has allotted to them, motor nerves must drive all substances to and sensation must judge the supply and demand. Nutrition must be in action the time and keep all parts well supplied with power to labor or a failure is sure to appear. We must ever remember the demands of nature on the lymphatics, liver and kidneys. They must work all the time or a confusion for lack in their duties will mark a cripple in some function of life over which they preside.

DUNGLINSON'S DEFINITION.

Dunglinson's scientific definition of the lymphatics is very extensive, comprehensive and right to the point for our use as doctors of Osteopathy. He describes the lymphatic glands as countless in number, universally distributed all through the human body, containing vitalized water and other fluids necessary to the support of animal life, running parallel with the venous system, and more abundantly there than in other locations of the body, at the same time discharging their contents into the veins while conveying the blood back to the heart from the whole system. Is it not reasonable to suppose that besides being nutrient centers, that they accumulate and pass water through the whole secretory and excretory systems of the body, in order to reduce nourishment to that degree from thick to thin, that it may easily pass through all tubes, ducts and vessels interested in distribution, as nourishment first, and renovation second, through the excretory ducts. The question arises whence cometh this water?

DANGERS OF DEAD SUBSTANCES.

This leads us back to the lungs as one of the great sources of which you have been informed under the head of "Lungs, Gases and Water." With this fountain of life saving water provided by nature to wash away impurities as they accumulate in our bodies, would it not be great stupidity in us to see a human being burn to death by the fires of fever, or die from asphyxia by allowing bad or dead lymph, albumen, or any substance to load down the powers of nature and keep the blood from being washed to normal purity? If so, let us go deeper into the study of the life-saving powers of the lymphatics. Do we not find in death that the lymphatics are dark, and in life they are healthy and red?

LYMPH CONTINUED.

What we meet with in all diseases is dead blood, stagnant lymph, and albumen in a semi-vital or dead and decomposing condition all through the lymphatics and other parts of the body, brain, lungs, kidneys, liver and fascia. The whole system is loaded with a confused mass of blood, that is mixed with much or little unhealthy substances, that should have been kept washed out by lymph. Stop and view the frog's superficial lymphatic glands; you see all parts move just as regular as the heart does; they are all in motion during life. For what purpose do they move? if not to carry the fluids to sustain by building up, while the excretory channels receive and pass out all that is of no further use to the body. Now we see this great system of supply is the source of construction and purity. If this be true we must keep them normal all the time or see confused nature in the form of disease, the list through. Thus we strike at the source of life and death when we go to the lymphatics.

With this fountain of life-saving water, provided by nature to wash away impurities as they accumulate in our bodies, would it not be great stupidity in us to see a human being burn to death by the fires of fever, or die from asphyxia, by allowing bad or dead lymph, albumen or any substance to load down the powers of nature to keep the blood washed to normal purity? If so let us go deeper in the study of the life-sustaining powers of the lymphatics.

NATURE'S SOLVENTS.

The brain flushes the nerves of the lymphatics first, and more than any other system of the body. No part is so small or remote that it is not in direct connection with some part or chain of the lymphatics. The doctor of Osteopathy has much to think about when he consults natural remedies, and how they are supplied and administered, and as disease is the effect of tardy deposits in some or all parts of the body, reason would bring us to hunt a solvent of such deposits, which hinder the natural motion of blood and other fluids in functional works, which are to keep the body pure from any substance that would check vital action. When we have searched and found that the lymphatics are almost the sole requisite of the body we then must admit that their use is equal to the abundant and universal supply of such glands. If we think and use a homely word and say that disease is only too much dirt in the wheels of life, then we will see that nature takes this method to wash out the dirt. As an application, pneumonia is too much dirt in the wheels of the lungs, if so we must wash out; no where can we go to a better place for water than to the lymphatics. Are they not like a fire company with nozzles in all windows ready to flush the burning house?

WHERE ARE THE LYMPHATICS SITUATED?

A student of life must take in all parts, and study their uses and relations to other parts and systems. We lay much stress on the uses of blood and the powers of the nerves, but have we any evidence that they are of more vital importance than the lymphatics? If not let us halt at this universal system of irrigation and study its great uses in sustaining animal life. Where are they situated in the body? Answer by, where are they not? No space is so small as to be out of connection with the lymphatics, with their nerves, secretory and excretory ducts. Thus the system of lymphatics is complete and universal in the whole body. After beholding the lymphatics distributed along all nerves, blood channels, muscles, glands and all organs of the body, from the brain to the soles of the feet, all loaded to fullness with watery liquids, we certainly can make but one conclusion as to their use, which would be to mingle with and carry out all impurities of the body, by first mixing with such substances and reducing them to that degree of fluids in fineness, that could pass through the smallest tubes of the excretory system, and by that method free the body from all deposits of either solids or fluids, and leave nourishment.

THE FAT AND LEAN.

A question: Why is he too fat and she only skin and bone, while a third is just right? If one is just right, why not all? If we get fat by a natural process why not reverse the process and stop at any desirable point in flesh size? I believe the law of life is simple and natural in both respects if wisely understood. Have we nerves of motion to carry food to all parts, organs, glands and muscles? Have we channels to convey to all? Have we fluids to suit all demands? Have we brain power equal to all force needed? Is blood formed sufficiently to fill all demands? Does that blood contain fat, water, muscle, skin, hair and all kinds to suit each division, organ, and nerve? If so and blood has builded too much flesh, can it not take that bulk away by returning blood to gas and other fluids? Can that which has been done be done again? If yes be the correct answer, then we should hope to return blood, fat, flesh and bone to gas and pass them away while in gaseous condition, and do away with all unnatural size or lack of size. I believe that it is natural to build and destroy all material form from the lowest animated being to the greatest rolling world. I believe no world could be constructed without strict obedience to a governing law, which gives size by addition and reduces that size by subtraction. Thus a fat man is builded by great addition, and if desired can be reduced by much subtraction, which is simply a rule of numbers. We multiply to enlarge, also subtract when we wish a reduction. Turn your eye for a time to the supply trains of nature. When the crop is abundant, the lading would be great, and when the seasons do not suit, the crops are short or shorter to no lading at all. Thus we have the fat man and the lean man. Is it not reasonable as a conclusion of the most exacting philosophy that the train of cars that can bring loads of stone, brick and mortar until a great bulk is formed, can also carry away until this bulk disappears in part or all? This being my conclusion I will say by many years of careful observation of the work of creating bodies and destroying the same, that to add to is the law of giving size, and to subtract from is the law of reduction. Both are natural, and both can be made practical in the reduction or addition of flesh, when found too great in quantity, or we can add to and give size to the starving muscle through the action of the motor and nutrient system conveyed to, and appropriated from the laboratory in which all bodily substances are formed. Thus the philosophy is absolute, and the sky is clear to proceed with addition and subtraction of flesh. I believe I am prepared to say at this time that I understand the nervous system well enough to direct the laboratory of nature and cause it through its skilled arts to unload, or reduce, he who is over-burdened with a super-abundance of flesh, and add to the scanty muscle a sufficiency to give power of comfortable locomotion and other forces, by opening the gate of the supply trains of nutrition.

CHAPTER VII.

THE DIAPHRAGM.

Investigation—A Struggle With Nature—Lesson of Cause and Effect—Something of Medical Etiquette—The Medical Doctor—An Explorer for Truth Must Be Independent—The Diaphragm Introduced—A Useful Study—Combatting Effect—Is Least Understood—A Case of Bilious Fever—A Demand on the Nerves— Danger of Compression—A Cause for Disease—Was a Mistake Made in the Creation—An Exploration—Result of Removal of Diaphragm—Sustaining Life in Principles—Law Applicable to Other Organs—Power of Diaphragm—Omentum.

INVESTIGATION.

Let us halt at the origin of the splanchnic and take a look. At this point we see the lower branches; sensation, motion, and nutrition, all slant above the diaphragm pointing to the solar plexus which sends off branches to pudic and sacral plexus of sensory system of nerves; just at the place to join the life giving ganglion of sacrum with orders from the brain to keep the process of blood forming in full motion all the time. A question arises, how is this motion supplied and from where? The answer is by the brain as nerve supply, heart as blood supply, all of which comes from above the diaphragm, to keep machinery in form and supplied with motion, that it may be able to generate chyle to send back to heart, to be formed into blood and thrown into arteries to build all parts as needed, and keep brain fed up to its normal supply of power generating needs. We see above the diaphragm, the lungs, heart and brain, the three sources of blood and nerve supply. All three are guarded by strong walls, that they may do their part in keeping up the life supply as far as blood and nerve force is required. But as they generate no blood nor nerve material, they must take the place of manufactories and purchase material from a foreign land, to be able to have an abundance all the time. We see nature has placed its manufactures above a given line in the breast, and grows the crude material below said line. Now as growth means motion and supply, we must combine in a friendly way, and conduct the force from above to the region below the septum or diaphragm, that we may use the powers as needed. This wall must and does have openings to let blood and nerves penetrate with supply and force to do the work of manufacturing.

A STRUGGLE WITH NATURE.

After all this has been done and a twist, pressure or obstructing fold should appear from any cause, would we not have a cut off of motion to return chyle, sensation to supply vitality, and venous motion to carry off arterial supply that has been driven from heart above? Have we not found the cause to stop all processes of life below diaphragm? In short, are we not in a condition to soon be in a complete state of stagnation? As soon as the arteries have filled the venous system, which is without sensation to return blood to the heart, then the heart can do nothing but wear out its energies trying to drive blood into a dead being below the diaphragm known as the venous system. It is dead until sensation reaches the vein from the sacral and pudic plexus.

LESSON OF CAUSE AND EFFECT.

Previous to all discoveries that have been made a demand for the usefulness of such discovery, is felt and talked of for years, centuries and cycles of time. Its discovery is an open question and free to all, because in this fact all are interested. That lack may be felt and spoken of by all agriculturists, and the inquiry directed to a better plow, a better sickle or mowing machine with which to reap standing grain. The thinker reduces his thoughts to practice, and cuts the grain, leaving it in such condition that a raker is needed to bunch it previous to binding.

His victory is heralded to the world as king of the harvest, and so accepted. The discoverer says, "I wish I could bunch that grain." He begins to reason from the great principle of cause and effect, and sleeps not until he has added to his already made discovery, an addition so ingeniously constructed that it will drop the grain in bunches ready for the binder. The discoverer stands by and sees in the form of a human being hands, arms and a band; he watches the motion then starts in to rustle with cause and effect again. He thinks and sweats day and night, and by the genius of thought produces a machine to bind the grain. By this time another suggestion arises, how to separate the wheat as the machine journeys in its cutting process. To his convictions nothing will solve this problem but mental action. He thinks and dreams of cause and effect. His mind seems to forget all the words of his mother tongue but cause and effect. He talks and preaches cause and effect in so many places that his associates begin to think he is mentally failing, and will soon be a subject for the asylum. He becomes disgusted with their lack of appreciation, seeks seclusion and formulates the desired addition and threshes the grain ready for the bag. He has solved the question and proved to his neighbors that the asylum was built for them, not for him. With cause and effect which is ever before the philosopher's eye, he ploughs the ocean regardless of the furious waves, he dreads not the storms on the seas, because he has so constructed a vessel with a resistance superior to the force of the lashing waves of the ocean, and the world scores him another victory. He opens his mouth and says by the law of cause and effect I will talk to my mother who is hundreds of miles away. He disturbs her rest by the rattling of a little electric bell in her room. Tremblingly the aged mother approaches the telephone and asks "Who is there?" And is answered, "It is me, Jimmie," and asks, "To whom am I talking?" She says "Mrs. Sarah Murphy." He says, "God bless you, mother; I am at Galveston, Texas, and you are in Boston, Mass." She laughs and cries with joy; he hears every emotion of her trembling voice. She says to him, "You have succeeded at last. I have never doubted your final success, notwithstanding the neighbors have annoyed me almost to death, telling me you would land in the asylum, because no man could talk so as to be heard 1000 miles away; his lungs, were too weak, and his tongue too short."

Now, friends, I have given you a long introductory foundation previous to giving you the cause of disease, with the philosophy that I have given upon cause and effect. I think it absolutely clear and the effect so unerring in its results, that with Pythagoras I can say "Eureka."

SOMETHING OF MEDICAL ETIQUETTE.

To know we have found a general cause for disease, one that will stand the heights and depths of direct and cross examinations, as given by the high courts of cool headed reason, has been the mental effort of all doctors and healers, since time began its record. They have had to treat disease as best they could, by such methods as customs had established as the best known for such diseases; notwithstanding their failures and the great mortality under such a system of treatment. They have not felt justified to go beyond the rules of symptomatology as adopted by their schools, with diagnosis, prognosis and treatment. Should they digress from the rules of the etiquette of their alma maters they would lose the brotherly love and support of the medical association to which they belong, under the belief that, "A bad name is as bad as death to a dog."

THE MEDICAL DOCTOR.

He says that in union there is safety, and resolves to stick to, live and do as his school has disciplined all its pupils, with this command, "The day thou eatest thereof, thou shalt surely die. Stick to the brotherhood."

AN EXPLORER FOR TRUTH MUST BE INDEPENDENT.

The explorer for truth must first declare his independence of all obligations or brotherhoods of any kind whatsoever. He must be free to think and reason. He must establish his observatory upon hills of his own; he must establish them above the imaginary high planes of rulers, kings, professors of schools of all kinds and denominations. He must be the Czar of his own mental empire, unencumbered with anything that will annoy while he makes his observations. I believe the reasons are so plain, so easily comprehended, the facts in its support so brilliant, that I will offer the same, though I be slaughtered on the altar of bigotry and intolerance. This philosophy is not intended for minds not thoroughly well posted by dissection and otherwise of the whole human anatomy. You must know its physiological laboratories and workings with the brain as the battery, the lungs as the source or machine that renovates the blood from all impurities, and the heart as the living engine or quarter-master, whose duty is to supply the commissaries with blood and other fluids to all divisions and sub-divisions of the human body, which is busily engaged producing material suited to the production of bone and muscle, and all other substances necessary to keep the machinery of life in full force and action.

Without this knowledge on the part of the reader, the words of this philosophy will fall as blanks before reaching his magazine of reason. Thus this is addressed to the independent man or woman that can, will and does reason.

THE DIAPHRAGM INTRODUCED.

At this point we will introduce the diaphragm, which separates the heart, lungs and brain from the organs of life that are limited to the abdomen and pelvis. A question arises at this point; what has the diaphragm to do with good or bad health? At this time we will analyze the diaphragm; we will examine its construction, and its uses; we will examine its openings through which blood passes both above and below. We will examine the opening through which food passes to stomach. We will carefully examine the passage or opening for nerve supply to the abdomen below, to run this great system of chemistry, which is producing the various kinds of substances necessary to the hard and soft parts of the body. We must know the nerve supply of the lymphatics, womb, liver, kidneys, pancreas, the generative organs, what they are, what they do, and what are demanded of them, before we are able to feed our own minds from the cup that contains the essence of reason as expressed from the tree of life.

A USEFUL STUDY.

The diaphragm surely gives much food to the one who would search for the great whys of disease as reported causes seem to be far back in the fogs of mystery. It may help us to arrive at some facts if we take each organ and division and make a full acquaintance of all its parts and uses before we combine it with others.

COMBATTING EFFECTS.

In all ages, the Doctor has for lack of knowledge of the true cause of diseases, combatted effects with his remedies. He treats pain with remedies to deaden pain; congestion to wash out overplus of blood that has been carried to parts or organs of the body by arteries of blood and channels of secretions and not taken up and passed out and off by the excretories. He sees the abnormal size and leaves the hunting of the cause that has given growth to such proportions and begins to seek rest and ease for his patient. Then he treats to reduce by medicine to carry the waste fluids to bowels, bladder and skin, with tonics to give strength and stimulants to increase the action of the heart in order to force local deposits to the general excretory system. At this time let the Osteopathic Doctor take a close hunt for any fold in muscles of the system that would cause a cut-off of the normal supply of blood or suspend the action of nerves whose office is to give power and action to the excretory system sufficient to keep the dead matter carried off as fast as it accumulates. Let us stop and acquaint ourselves with the true condition of the diaphragm. It must be normal in place, as it is so situated that it will admit of no abnormality. It must be kept stretched, just as Nature arranged that it should, like a drum-head. It is attached all around to the chest, though it crosses five or six ribs on its descent from the seventh rib to the sternum at the lower point and down to fourth lumbar vertebra. It is a continuous slanting floor, above bowels and abdominal organs, and below heart and lungs. It must, by all reason, be kept normal in tightness at all places, without a fold or wrinkle, that could press the aorta, nerves, œsophagus, or anything that contributes to the supply or circulation of any vital substance. Now can there be any move in spine or ribs that would or could change the normal shape of the diaphragm? If so, where and why?

IS LEAST UNDERSTOOD.

The diaphragm is possibly the least understood as being the cause of more diseases, when its supports are not all in line and normal position, than any other part of the body. It has many openings through which nerves, blood and food pass while going from chest to all parts below. It begins at the lower end of the breast-bone and crosses to ribs back and down, in a slanting direction to the third or fourth lumbar vertebra. Like an apron, it holds all that is above it up, such as heart and lungs, and is the fence that divides the organs of the abdomen from the chest. Below it are the stomach, bowels, liver, spleen, kidneys, pancreas, womb, bladder; also the great system of lymphatics of the whole blood and nerve supply of the organs and systems of nutrition and life supply. All parts of the body have a direct or indirect connection with this great separating muscle. It assists in breathing, in all animals, when normal, and when prolapsed by the falling in and down of any of the five or six ribs by which it is supported in place, then we suffer from the effects of suspended normal arterial supply, and venous stagnation below diaphragm. The aorta meets resistance as it goes down with blood to nourish, and the vein as it goes back with impurities contained in venous blood, also meets an obstruction at the diaphragm, as it returns to the heart through the vena cava, because of the packing of a fallen diaphragm on and about the blood vessels that must not be obstructed. Thus heart trouble, lung disease, brain, liver, womb, tumors of the abdomen and through the list of effects can be traced to the diaphragm as the cause.

I am strongly impressed that the diaphragm has much to do in keeping all the machinery and organs of life in a healthy condition, and will try and give some of the reasons why, as I now understand them. First, it is found to be wisely located just below the heart and lungs; one being the engine of the blood, and the other is the engine of the air. This strong wall holds all substances or other bodies away from any chance to press on either engine, while performing their parts in the economy of life. Each engine has a sacred duty to perform under the penal law of death to itself and all other divisions of the whole being, man. If it should neglect its work of which it is a vital part, should we take down this wall and allow the liver, stomach and spleen to occupy any of the places allotted to these engines of life, a confusion would surely be the result; ability of the heart to force blood to the lungs would be overcome and cause trouble.

A CASE OF BILIOUS FEVER.

Suppose we take a few diseases and submit them to the crucial ordeal of reason, and see if we do, or can find any one of the climatic fevers that appear with its full list of symptoms and have no assistance from an irritated diaphragm. For example take a case of common bilious fever of North America. It generally begins with a tired and sore feeling of limbs and muscles, pain in spine, head, and lumbar region. At this point of our inquiry we are left in an open sea of mystery and conjecture as to cause. One says, "malaria," and goes no farther, gives a name and stops. If you ask for the cause of such torturous pain in head and back, with fever and vomiting, he will tell you that the very best authorities agree that the cause is malaria, with its peculiar diagnostic tendency to affect the brain, spine and stomach, and administers quinine and leaves, thinking he has said and done all.

Reason would lead seekers for cause of the pain above located to remember that all blood passes first as chyme up to heart and lungs, directly through the diaphragm, conducted through the thoracic duct, first to heart, thence to lungs, at the same time rivers of blood are pouring into the heart from all of the system. Much of it very impure, from diseased or stale blood. Much of the chyle is dead before it enters the great thoracic duct and goes to the lungs without enough pure blood to sustain life. Then disease appears.

As a cut-off the diaphragm, when dropped front and down, and across the aorta and vena cava by a lowering of the ribs, on both sides of the spine; it would be a complete pressure over cœlic axis, with liver supply, renal, pelvic, to a complete abdominal stoppage. Then we have over-due blood for other parts to send off dead corpuscles by asphyxia, with no hope that it can sustain life and health of the parts for which it was designed. Thus we know that nature would not be true to its own laws, if it would do good work with bad material.

A DEMAND ON THE NERVES.

Why not reason on the broad scale of known fact, and give the "why" he or she has complete prostration when all systems are wholly cut off from a chance to move and execute such duties as nature has allotted to them. Motor nerves must drive all substances to, and sensation must judge the supply and demand. Nutrition must be in action all the time and keep all parts well supplied or a failure is sure to appear. We must ever remember the demands of nature on the lymphatics, liver and kidneys, that nerves work all the time or a confusion for lack in their duties will mark a cripple in some function of life over which they preside.

DANGER OF COMPRESSION.

At this time we see by all systems of reason that no delay in passage of food or blood, can be tolerated at the diaphragm, because any irritation is bound to cause muscular contraction and impede the natural flow of blood, first through the abdominal aorta, and even to a temporary, partial or complete stoppage of arterial supply to the abdomen. Or the vena cava may be so pressed as to completely stop the return of venous blood from the stomach, kidneys, bowels and all other organs, such as the lymphatics, pancreas, fascia, cellular membranes, nerve centers, ganglionic and all systems of supply of organs of life found in the abdomen. Thus by pressure, stricture or contraction to the passage of blood can be stopped, either above or below the diaphragm, and be the cause of blood being detained long enough to die from asphyxia, and be left in the body of all organs below the diaphragm.

A CAUSE FOR DISEASE.

Thus you see a cause for Bright's disease of kidneys, disease of womb, ovaries, jaundice, dysentery, leucorrhœa, painful monthlies, spasms, dyspepsia, and on through the whole list of diseases now booked as "causes unknown," and treated by the rule of "cut and try." We do know that all blood for use of the whole system below the twelfth dorsal vertebra does pass through the diaphragm, and all nerve supply, also passes through the diaphragm and spinal column for limb and life. This being a known fact, we have only to use reason to know that an unhealthy condition of the diaphragm is bound to be followed by many diseases. A list of questions arise at this point with the inquirers that must and can be answered every time by reason only. The diaphragm is a musculo-fibrinous organ and depends for blood and nerve supply above its own location, and that supply must be given freely and pure for nerve and blood or we will have a diseased organ to start with; then we may find a universal atrophy or œdema, which would, besides its own deformity not be able to rise and fall, to assist the lungs to mix air with blood to purify venous blood, as it is carried to the lungs to throw off impurities and take on oxygen previous to returning to the heart, to be sent off as nourishment for the system. It is only in keeping with reason that without a healthy diaphragm both in its form and action, disease is bound to be the result. A question from our side of the argument is: How can a carpenter build a good house out of rotten, twisted or warped wood? If he can, then we can hope to be healthy with diseased blood, but if we must have good material in building, then we should form our thoughts to suit the heads of inspectors, and inspect the passage of blood through the diaphragm, pleury, pericardium and the fascia, superficial, deep and universal. Disease is just as liable to begin its work in the fascia and epithelium as any other place. Thus the necessity of pure blood and healthy fascia, because all functions are equally responsible for good and bad results.

WAS A MISTAKE MADE IN THE CREATION?

At a given period of time the Lord said, "Let us make man." After He had made him He examined him, and pronounced him good, and not only good, but very good. Did He know what good was? Had He the skill to be a competent judge? If He was perfectly competent to judge skilled arts His approval of the work when done was the fiat of mental competency backed by perfection. Since that architect and skilled mechanic has finished man and given him dominion over the fowls of the air, the beast of the field and fishes of the sea, hasn't that person, being or superstructure proven to us that God, the creator of all things, has armed him with strength, with the mind and machinery to direct and execute? This being demonstrated and leaving us without a doubt as to its perfection, are we not admonished by all that is good and great to enter upon a minute examination of all the parts belonging to this being; acquaint ourselves with their uses and all the designs for which the whole being was created. If we are honestly interested with the acquaintance of the forms and uses of the parts in detail by close and thorough examination of the material, its form and object of its form, from whence this substance is obtained; how it is produced and sustained through life in kind and form. How it is moved, where it gets its power, and for what object does it move? A demand for a crucial examination of the skull, the heart, lungs, of the chest, the stomach, liver and other organs of the abdomen is made. The septum of the brain, the pericardium of the chest—the diaphragm of the abdomen which is a dividing septum between the abdomen and chest. In this examination we must know the reasons why any organs, vessel or any other substance is located at a given place. We must run with all the rivers of blood that travel through the system.

AN EXPLORATION.

We must start our exploring boat with the aorta, and float with this vital current; see the captain as he unloads supplies for the diaphragm and all that is under it. We must follow him and see what branch of this river will lead to a little or great toe, or to the terminals of the whole foot. We must pass through the waters of the dead sea by the way of the vena cava, and observe the boats loaded with exhausted and worn out blood, as it is poured in and channeled back to the heart, with all below the diaphragm. Carefully watch the emptying of the vena azygos major and minor, with the veins of the arms and head all being poured in from little or great rivers to the vena innominate on their way to the great hospital of life and nourishment; whose quarter-master is the heart; whose finishing mechanic is the lung. Having acquainted ourselves with the forms and locations of this great personality we are ready at this time after examination, and found worthy and well qualified to enter into a higher class in which we can obtain an acquaintance with the physiological workings separately and conjoined of the whole being. At this place we become acquainted with the hows and whys of the production of blood, bone and all elements found in them, necessary to sustain sensation, motion, nutrition, voluntary and involuntary action of the nerve system. The hows and whys of the lymphatics, the life sustaining powers of the brain, heart, lungs, and all the abdominal system, with their various actions and uses, from the lowest cellular membrane to the highest organ of the body.

RESULT OF REMOVAL OF DIAPHRAGM.

When we consult the form of the cross-bar that divides the body in two conjoined divisions and reason on its use, we arrive at the fact that the heart and lungs must have ample space or room to suit their actions while performing their functions. At this time a question comes up: What effect would follow the removal of the fence between heart, lungs and brain, above that dividing muscle, and the machinery that is situated below said cross-bar? We see at a glance that we would meet failure to the extent of the infringement on demanded room for normal work of heart to deliver below lungs to prepare blood, and the brain to pass nerve power to either engine above, and all organs below the diaphragm.

SUSTAINING LIFE PRINCIPLES.

The life of the living tree is with the bark and superficial fascia which lies between the bark of the body of the tree, its periostium. The remainder of the tree takes the position or place of secreting. Its excretory system is first upwards from the surface of the ground, and washes out frozen impurities in the spring, after which it secretes and conveys to the ground through the trunk of the tree to the roots which is like unto the placenta attached to mother earth, qualifying all substances of constructing fiber and leaf, of that part of the tree above the ground. Each year produces a new tree which is seen and known by circular rings called annular growths. That growth which was completed last year is now a stale being of the past and has no vital action of itself. But like all stale beings its process is a life of another order, and dependent upon the fascia for its life and cellular action which lies under the bark, for its own existence as a living tree. It can only act as a chemical laboratory and furnish crude material which is taken up by the superficial fascia and conveyed up to the lungs, and exchanges dead for living matter, to receive and return to all parts of the tree, keeping up vital formation. With frost its vital process ceases through the winter season until mother earth stimulates the placenta, and starts the growth of a new being, which is developed and placed in form on the old trunk. Thus you see everything of animal growth as we would call them, is a new being, and becomes a part of the next being or growth formed.

STALE LIFE.

Should this form of vitality cease with the tree another principle which we call stale life takes possession and constructs another tree which is just the reverse of the living tree, and builds a tree after its own power of formulation from the dead matter, to which it imparts a principle of stale life, which life produces mushrooms, frogstools and other peculiar forms of stale beings, from this form of growth.

Thus we are prepared to reason that blood when ligated and retained in that condition of dead corpuscles, and no longer able to support animal life, can form a zoophyte and all the forms peculiar to the great law of association, as tumefactions of the lymphatics, pancreas, liver, kidneys, uterus, with all the glandular system, be they lymphatics, cellular, ganglia or any other parts of the body susceptible of such growths, below the diaphragm. Thus we can account for tubercles of the abdomen and all organs therein found.

LAW APPLICABLE TO OTHER ORGANS.

This same law is equally applicable to the heart, lungs, the brain, tissues, glands, fascia and all substances capable of receiving without the ability to excrete stale substances.

As œdema marks the first tardiness of fluids we have the beginning step which will lead from miliary tuberculosis to the largest known forms of tubercles, which is the effect of the active principles of stale life or the life of dead matter.

POWER OF DIAPHRAGM.

At this point we will draw the attention of the reader to the fact that the diaphragm can contract and suspend the passage of blood and produce all the stagnant changes from start to completed deadly tubercle. Also the cancer, the wen, glandular thickening of neck, face, scalp, fascia and all substances found above the diaphragm. In this stale life we have a compass that will lead us as explorers from the North star, to the South pole, the rising sun of reason, and the evening dews of eternity. This diaphragm says: "By me you live and by me you die. I hold in my hand the powers of life and death, acquaint now thyself with me and be at ease."

OMENTUM.

The truth of the presentation of facts should be the principle object of every person who takes his pen with a view to give the reasons why certain witnesses' testimony are indispensable to establish supposable or known truths. This being the case I have summoned before this court of inquiry an important witness. He has now taken the oath to tell the truth, the whole truth and nothing but the truth, of the case before this court. His name is the Great Omentum. Mr. Omentum, state if you know of any reason why or how by irritation from a misplacement of your body or any of its attachments to or about the diaphragm, the spine, stomach or other places that could cause irritation and thickening by congestion of your own body to such degree as to impede the flow of arterial or venous blood, over whose position you occupy much space from the diaphragm downward? State what effect a falling down of the eleventh and twelfth ribs on both sides of the spine with their cartilaginous points turned inward and down; if they should draw the diaphragm down and across your body? What would be the effect on circulation of the blood, and other fluids on the kidneys and other organs of the abdomen and pelvis? Would it not be the foundation for destructive congestion, and abnormal growth? State if you know if any such ligation would cause swelling by retention of blood in the spleen, liver, kidneys or other organs of the abdomen and pelvis? Would it be reasonable to suppose that you could perform your functions in office with any irritating condition caused by prolapses of diaphragm? Would not an irritation of your attachment to the diaphragm, spine or stomach be great enough to impede the blood on its passage through the aorta to the abdomen, or impede the flow of blood back and through the diaphragm? If so state how and why?

CHAPTER VIII.

LIVER, BOWELS AND KIDNEYS.

Gender of the Liver—Productions of the Liver—A Hope for the
Afflicted—Evidences of Truth—Loaded With Ignorance—Lack of
Knowledge of the Kidney—How a Purgative Acts—Flux—Bloody
Dysentery—Flux More Fully Described—Osteopathic Remedies—
Medical Remedies—More of the Osteopathic Remedy.

GENDER OF THE LIVER.

Let us abruptly assume that the liver is the abiding placenta of all
animated beings. If this position be true we are warranted and
justified in the conclusion that the germs necessary to form blood
vessels and other parts of the body must look to the liver for the
fluids in which they would expect to construct in form and size. It
seems to be nature's chemical laboratory, in which are prepared by
receiving chemical qualities and quantities to suit the formation of
hard and soft substances, which are to become the parts and the
whole of any organ, gland, muscle, nerve, cell, veins and arteries. In
evidence of the probability of the truth of this position, we will draw
your attention, first to its central location between the sacral and
cerebral nerve centers. There it lies between the "stomach" the vessel
which receives all material previous to being manipulated for all
nutrient purposes, and the heart, the great receiving and distributing
quarter-master of all animal life. It supplies squads, sections,
companies, regiments, battalions, brigades and divisions—to the
whole army, and all parts that are dependent upon the nutrient
system.

PRODUCTIONS OF THE LIVER.

The liver seems to be able to qualify by calling to itself all substances
necessary to produce gall. Its communications with all parts of the
body is direct, circuitous, universal and absolute. If pure it produces
healthy gall and other substances, and in fact when healthy itself all
other fluids are considered to be pure, at which time we are

supposed to enjoy good health and universal bodily comfort. With a diseased liver we have perverted action which possibly accounts for impure and unhealthy deposits in the nasal passage and other parts of the body in their own peculiar form. Polypus of the nose, tumefaction of lungs, lymphatics, liver, kidneys, uterus, and even the brain itself. Suppose such deposits, composed of albumen and fibrin, prepared in the liver should be deposited in the lining membranes of veins leading to the heart, and by some other chemical action this accumulated mass should come loose from the veins, would we not expect what is commonly called clots enter the heart, and shut off the arteries, supplying the lungs, stop the further circulation of blood and cause instantaneous death called heart failure, apoplexy and so on? Is it not reasonable to suppose that under those deposits that softening of arteries has its beginning, which results in aneurisms and death by rupture of such abnormally formed arteries? Are the lungs not liable to receive such deposits and form tubercles to such proportions as to become living zoophytes capable of covering all of the mucous membrane of the lungs, air passages and cells, and establish a perpetual dwelling of zoophytes and absorb to themselves for their own maintenance and existence, blood and nourishment of the whole body unto death? This being the result of one chemical action of the body and all by and from nature, is it not reasonable to suppose that the provision by nature is ready to produce of itself the chemicals of kind, quality and quantity equal to the destruction of this enemy of life?

A HOPE FOR THE AFFLICTED.

I think before all diseases pass the zenith, after which the decline is beyond the vital rally, they are curable by the genius of nature's own remedies, and believe the truths of this conclusion have been supported abundantly by daily demonstrations. I believe there is hope for the consumptive equal to one-half if not greater when taken in proper time, which is at any period of the disease, previous to breaking down by ulceration or otherwise, lung tissue, and even after this period, hope is not altogether lost.

EVIDENCES OF TRUTH.

Nature and good sense are terms that mean much to persons who are used to set aside all else for facts. A fact may and often does stay before our eyes for all time powerful in truth, but we heed not its lessons. Instances, at least a few, would not be amiss at this time. Electricity, the most powerful force known, was never able with all its works to get the attention of man's thoughts, more than to call it thunder and lightning, and let it pass from his mind from time to time, till brighter ages woke up a Franklin, Edison, Morse and others who heeded its useful lessons enough to make application of its powers for its force and speed. By the results obtained, they and others have used its powers and gotten truths as rewards, that they did not know even existed in or out of electricity or in any of the store-houses of all nature. But as the winds of time have blown open a few leaves of nature's book, and their brilliant pages and useful lessons have found a lodging place in such persons as were endowed with wisdom to see, and patience to persevere, by their energy and wisdom to-day we have many pages to add to our books of useful knowledge. We can now talk around and all over the earth by the power of the dreaded thunder and lightning. By it we travel, by it we see at night, by it we search on land and sea for friend or foe; in fact, it is dreaded no more but sought, used and loved by all who know of its uses in civil life. Thus our enemy has become our footstool. By the speed of man's ability we know and use the comforts that nature holds in store for us until we call for and use them.

Other and just as useful questions as electricity await our attention. Parts and uses of the human body, to-day are to us as little understood as electricity was at any time. The lung to-day is an unknown mystery, as to what its power and uses are; we only know that air goes in and out of the lungs; farther than that we are at sea. We have just as little knowledge of the heart as the lungs, we find a hollow fibrinous tank receiving and discharging blood; we are not prepared to say whether the corpuscle is formed in the heart or not; all else is conjectural and speculative on the subject the corpuscle. We see channels leading to and from it, to and from all parts of the body, muscles and glands. We know it moves when we are alive, we know it is silent in death.

LOADED WITH IGNORANCE.

We pass from there to the liver loaded down with ignorance, from what we know, cannot tell whether it is male or female, we simply know its size, location and something of its form and action, but nothing beyond conjecture. It stands to-day one of the wonders to him that tries to reason.

LACK OF KNOWLEDGE OF THE KIDNEY.

We will leave this organ of many pounds with an open confession of our ignorance and take up the kidney. At what time was the man and woman born that knew and left on record a true and reliable knowledge of the renal capsule. We do not know whether that is the organ that makes our teeth, our hair or generates a powerful acid by which lime is kept in solution, so as not to form stones and such deposits.

HOW A PURGATIVE ACTS.

Nature's method is simple and easily comprehended in delivering purgative medicines, with their softening powers to dry constipated fecal matter. For instance: We would give a purgative in the shape of salts, rhubarb, calomel and other substances of choice. The first question of the physician is how is this to pass through so densely packed substance or fecal matter which is in the bowels? At this time we will be short in the statement. The purgative poisons are taken up by the the secretions conveyed to the lymphatics. To soften and wash out is the object of nature. The lymphatics begin the work of washing out by starting action of the excretories and furnishes the water to soften, which is injected into the bowels from the mouth to the extremities by a system of salivation.

FLUX (BLOODY DYSENTERY.)

Flux is common in all temperate climates. It generally shows its true nature as dysentery after a few hours of tiresome feeling, aching in head, back and bowels. At first nothing is felt or thought of more than a few movements of the bowels than is common for each day. Some pain and griping are felt with increase at each stool, until a chilly feeling is felt all over the body, with violent pains in lower bowels, with pressing desire to go to stool, and during and after passage of stool a feeling that there is still something in the bowels that must pass. Soon that down pressure partially subsides, and on examination of passage a quantity of blood is seen which shows the case is bloody flux, as the disease is called and known in the southern states of North America, or bloody dysentery in the more northern states. It generally subsides by the use of family remedies, such as sedatives, astringents, and palliative diets. But the severity in other cases increases and the discharges have more blood, greater pain, mixed with gelatinous substance even to mucous membrane of bowels, high fever all over except abdomen, which is quite cold to the hand. Back, head and limbs suffer much with heat and pain, and much nausea is felt at all motions of bowels. Bowels change from cold to hot, even to 104, at which time all symptoms point to inflammation of the bowels. The colon in particular, at which time discharge grows black, frothy and very offensive from decomposition of blood. Soon collapse and death close out the case, notwithstanding the very best skill has been employed to save the life of the patient. The doctor has tried to stop pain by opiates and other sedatives, tried to check bowels with astringents, used tonics and stimulants, but all have failed, the patient is dead.

HOW DOES THE OSTEOPATH CURE?

But the question for the Osteopath is: At what point would you work to suppress the sensation of the colon and permit veins to open and allow blood to return to heart? Does irritation of a sensory nerve cause vein to contract and refuse blood to complete circuit from and to the heart? Does flux begin with the sensory nerves of bowels? If so, reduce sensation at all points connecting with bowels, stop all overplus, keep veins free and open from cutaneous to deep sensory ganglion of whole spine and abdomen. Remember the fascia is what suffers and dies in all cases of death by bowels and lungs. Thus the nerves of all the fascia of bowels and abdomen must work or you may lose all cases of flux, for in the fascia exists much of the soothing and vital qualities of nature. Guard it well, so it can work to repair all losses or death will begin in fascia and through pass it to the whole system.

FLUX MORE FULLY DESCRIBED.

"Bloody flux" is a flow of blood with other fluids from the mucous membrane of the bowels. A disease generally of the summer and fall seasons, and is more abundant south than north of latitude 40° of North America. It is so well known in this country by its ravages that to describe it is almost useless, as bloody fluids pass from bowels in all cases.

We reason that the veins have contracted by nerve irritation and fail to convey blood to heart on normal time. By which delay decomposition does its work. Thus a cause is seen for excreting fluids by motor action of bowels, when supplied by the excretory system.

OSTEOPATHIC REMEDIES.

An Osteopath to successfully treat flux or bloody dysentery must reason and address his attention first to the soreness and irritation of bowels, which he finds suffering with œdema of mucous membrane of all the glands and blood vessels belonging to the lower bowels. As quiet is the first thing desired, he will direct his attention to the sensory nerves of the colon and small intestines, in order to reduce the resistance of the veins and diminish the arterial action. When he has diminished sensation of the veins of the bowels, the arterial force completes its circuit through the veins back to the heart, with much less arterial action, because venous resistance has ceased and the circuit is normal, and healthy action is the result.

MEDICAL REMEDIES.

The medicine man addresses his remedies first to the misery, with the desire to relax the nerves and overcome pain, and obtains this result through some class of opiates. After a short rest he addresses his attention to the motor action of the heart, with the view of giving arteries greater power to force arterial blood through all obstructions, and tries to stop all excretory wastings by the use of astringents combined with sedatives and soothing fluids.

MORE OF THE OSTEOPATHIC REMEDY.

The Osteopath will govern sensory and motor nerves by digital suspension of the abnormal irritability of the sensory nerves on the various parts of the spine as indicated by the disease.

He uses no injections for the bowels for the reason that the necessary fluids naturally flow into the bowels to lubricate and quiet, and proceed at once to repair all irritated surfaces, which is abundantly supplied by nature from the mouth of the sphincter ani, without which forethought and preparation, nature's God will prove his incompetency for the great battle of life.

You administer medicines from the chemistry of the arts by mouth, injection and otherwise. We adjust the machinery and depend upon nature's chemical laboratory for all elements necessary to repair, give ease and comfort, while nature's corpuscles do all the work necessary.

CHAPTER IX.

THE BLOOD.

Uses for Fluids—Blood an Unknown Fluid—Harvey Only Reached the Banks of the River of Life—Blood Is Systematically Furnished—Fatality of Ignorance—To Find the Cause Must Be Honest—Following Arteries and Nerves—Feeding the Nerves—The Blood on Its Journey—Powers Necessary to Move Blood—Venous Blood Suspended.

USES FOR FLUIDS.

If a thousand kinds of fluids exist in our bodies a thousand uses require their help, or they would not appear. Thus to know how and why they help in the economy of life is the study of he who acts only when he knows at what places each must appear, and fill the part and use for which it is designed. If the demand for a substance is absolute its chance to act and answer that call and obey such command must not be hindered while in preparation, nor on its journey to local destination, for by its power all action may depend. Thus blood, albumen, gall, acids, alkalies, oils, brain fluid and other substances formed by associations while in physiological processes of formation must be on time in place and measured abundantly, that the biogenic laws of nature can have full power with time to act, and material in abundance and of kinds to suit. Thus all things else may be in place in ample quantities and fail because the power is withheld and no action for want of brain fluids with its power to vivify all animated nature which have followed any fluid found in the body, and followed it from formation to use and exhaustion step by step until he knows what form a union with one or many kinds. Thus we can do no more than feed and trust the laws of life as nature gives them to man. We must arrange our bodies in such true lines that ample nature can select and associate by its definite measures, weights and choices of kinds, that which can make all fluids needed for our bodily uses, from the crude blood to the active flames of life, as seen when marshalled for the duties of that stands and obey the edicts of the mind of the infinite.

BLOOD AN UNKNOWN FLUID.

Blood is an unknown red or black fluid, found inside of the human body, in tubes, channels or tunnels. What it is, how it is made, and what it does after it leaves the heart in the arteries, before it returns to the heart through the veins, is one of the mysteries of animal life. It has been tried to be analyzed to know of what it is composed, and when done, we know but little more of what it really is, than we know what sulphur is made of. We know it is a colored fluid, and it is in all parts of the flesh and bone. We know it builds up heaps of flesh, but how, is the question that leads us to honor the unknowable law of life, by which it does the work of its mysterious construction of all forms found in the parts of man. In all our efforts to learn what it is, what it is made of, and what enters it as life and gives it the building powers with that intelligence it displays in building, that we see in daily observation, is to us such an incomprehensible wonder, that with the "sacred writers" we are constrained to say, Great is the mystery of "Godliness." I dislike to say we know but very little about the blood, "in fact, nothing at all," but such is the truth under oath. We cannot make one drop of blood because of our ignorance of the laws of its production. If we knew what its components were, we would soon build large machinery, make and have blood for sale in quantities to suit the purchaser. But alas! we cannot with all the combined intelligence of man, make one drop of blood, because we do not know what it is. Then, as its production is by the skill of a foreigner whose education has grown to suit the work, we must silently sit by and willingly receive the work when handed out for use by the producer. At this point I will say that an intelligent Osteopath is willing to be governed by the immutable laws of nature, and feel that he is justified to pass the fluid on from place to place and trust results.

HARVEY ONLY REACHED THE BANKS OF THE RIVER OF LIFE.

When Harvey solved by his powers of reason a knowledge of the circulation of the blood, he only reached the banks of the river of life. He saw that the heads and mouths of the rivers of blood begin and end in the heart, to do the mysterious works of constructing man.

Then he went into camp and left this compound for other minds to speculate on, of the how it was made, of what composed, and how it became a medium of life which sustains all beings. He saw the genius of nature had written its wisdom and will of life, by the red ink of all truth.

BLOOD IS SYSTEMATICALLY FURNISHED.

Blood is systematically furnished from the heart to all divisions of our bodies. When we go any course from the heart we will find one or more arteries leaving heart. If we go toward the head, we find caroted, cervical and vertebral arteries in pairs, large enough to supply blood abundantly for bone, brain, and muscle. That blood builds all the brain, all the bone, nerves, muscles, glands, membranes, fascia and skin. Then we see wisdom just as much in the venous system, as in the arterial. Thus the arteries supply all demands, and the veins carry away all waste material, with returning blood of veins. We find building and healthy renovation are united in a perpetual effort to construct and sustain purity. In these two are the facts and truths of life and health. If we go to any other part or organ of the body, we find just the same law of supply, arteries first, then renovation, beginning with the veins. The rule of artery and vein is universal in all living beings, and the Osteopath must know that, and abide by its rulings, or he will not succeed as a healer. Place him in open combat with fevers of winter or summer and he saves, or loses, his patients, just in proportion to his ability to sustain the artery to feed, and the veins to purify by taking away the dead substances before they ferment, in the lymphatics and cellular system. He shows just the same stupidity and ignorance of support from arteries and purity by the veins when he fails to cure erysipelas, flux, pneumonia, croup, scarlet fever, diphtheria, measles, mumps, rheumatism, and on to all diseases of climate and seasons.

FATALITY OF IGNORANCE.

It is ignorance and inattention to the arteries to supply and the veins to carry away all deposits before they form tumors in lungs, abdomen or any part of the system. Thus man's ignorance of how and why the blood renovates and why tumors are formed, has allowed the knife to be found in the belts of so many doctors to-day. On this law Osteopathy has successfully stood and cured more than any school of cures, and has sustained all its diplomates financially and otherwise. I write this article on blood for the student of Osteopathy. I want him to put nature to a test of its merit, and know if it is a law equal to all demands. If not, he is very much and seriously limited when he goes into war with diseases. What is to be understood by "Disease?"[5]

When we use the word "disease," we mean anything that makes an unnatural showing in the body by pain, overgrowth of muscle; gland; organ; physical pain; numbness; heat; cold; or anything that we find not necessary to life and comfort. I have no wish to rob surgery of its useful claims, and its scientific merits to suffering man and beast. Such is not my object, but to place the Osteopath's eye of reason on the hunt of the great whys that the knife is useful at all, I am sure it comes often to remove growths and diseased flesh and bone that have gotten so by man's ignorance of a few great truths. 1st, If blood is allowed to be taken to a gland or organ, and not taken away in due time the accumulation will become bulky enough to stop the excretory nerves and cause local paralysis; then the nutrient nerves proceed to construct tumors, and on and on until there is no relief but the knife or death. Had this blood not been conveyed there, it would not be there at all, either in bulk or less quantities. Had it simply done its work and passed on we could have no material to grow such abnormal beings. If a tumefaction appears in one side, and not in the other, why so? and why is there no growth in one side the same as the other? It takes no great effort of mind to see that the veins did not receive and carry off the blood, and a growth was natural, as the condition could not do otherwise and be true to nature. Thus man's ignorance has made a condition for the knife. Had he taken the hint and let the blood pass on when its work was done, he would not have to witness the guillotine of death to his patients, whose early pains told him a renal vein or some vessel below the diaphragm was ligated by an impacted colon, or a few ribs pulling and bringing diaphragm down across vena cava and thoracic duct and causing excitement or paralysis of solar plexus, or any other nerves that pass through diaphragm with blood to and from heart and lungs.

TO FIND THE CAUSE.

How to find causes of diseases or where a hindrance is located that stops blood is a great mental worry to the Osteopath when he is called to treat a patient. The patient tells him "where he hurts," how much "he hurts," how long "he has hurt," how hot or cold he is. The doctor puts this symptom and that symptom in a column, adds them up according to the latest books on symptomatology, finally he is able to guess at some name to call the disease. Then he proceeds and treats as his pap's father heard his granny say their old family doctor treated "them sort of diseases in North Carolina." An Osteopath feels bad to have to hunt cause for diseases, and not know how to start out to find the mechanical cause. He feels that the people expect more than guessing of an Osteopath. He feels that he must put his hand on the cause and prove what he says by what he does, that he will not get off by the feeble minded trash of stale habits that go with doctors of medicine, and by his knowledge he must show his ability to go beyond the musty bread of symptomatology and water his patients made, from the cider of the ripe apples from the tree of knowledge.

MUST BE HONEST.

An Osteopath should be a clear-headed, conscientious, truth loving man, and never speak until he knows he has found and can demonstrate the truth he claims to know.

FOLLOWING ARTERIES AND NERVES.

I understand anatomy and physiology after fifty years casual and close attention, the last twenty years being very continued and close attention to what has been said, by all the best writers whom I have perused, many of whom are considered standard guides for the student and practitioner to be governed by. I have dissected and witnessed the very best anatomists that the world affords dissect. I have followed the knife after arteries through the whole distribution of blood of arterial systems, to the great and small vessels, until the lenses of the most powerful microscopes seemed to exhaust their ability to perceive the termination of the artery; with the same care following the knife and microscope from nerve center to terminals of the large to the infinitely small fibers around which those fine nerve vines entwine. First like a bean entwining by way of the right around and up continuing to the right, and then turn my microscope to the entwining of another set of nerves which is to the left universally as the hop. Those nerves are solid, cylindrical and stratified in form, with many leading from the lymphatics to the artery, and to the red and white muscles, fascia, cellular-membrane, striated and unstriated organs, all connecting to and traveling with the artery, and continuing with it through its whole circuit from start to terminals.

FEEDING THE NERVES.

Like a thirsty herd of camels, the whole nerve system, sensory, motor, nutrient, voluntary and involuntary; this herd of sappers or hungry nerves seems to be in sufficient quantities and numbers to consume all blood and cause the philosopher to ask the question: "Is not the labor of the artery complete when it has fed the hungry nerves?" Is he not justified in the conclusion that the nerves do gestate and send forth all substances that are applied by nature in the construction of man? If this philosophy be true, then he who arms himself for the battles of Osteopathy when combating diseases, has a guide and a light whereby he can land safely in port from every voyage.

THE BLOOD ON ITS JOURNEY.

Turn the eye of reason to the heart and observe the blood start on its journey. It leaves in great haste and never stops even in the smaller arteries. It is all in motion and very quick and powerful at all places. Its motion indicates no evidence of construction even supposable during such time, but we can find in the lymphatics, cells or pockets, motion slow enough to suppose that in such cells, living beings can be formed and carried to their places by the lymphatics for the purposes they must fill, as bone, or muscle. Let us reason that blood has a great and universal duty to perform, if it constructs, nourishes, and keeps the whole nerve system normal in form and function.

POWERS NECESSARY TO MOVE BLOOD.

As blood and other fluids of life are ponderable bodies of different consistences, and are moved through the system to construct, purify, vitalize and furnish power necessary to keep the machinery in action, we must reason on the different powers necessary to move those bodies through arteries, veins, ducts, over nerves, spongy membranes, fascia, muscles, ligaments, glands and skin; and judge from their unequal density, and adjust force to meet the demand according to kinds, to be sent to and from all parts.

VENOUS BLOOD SUSPENDED.

Suppose venous blood to be suspended by cold or other causes in the lungs to the amount of œdema of the fascia, another mental look would see the nerves of the fascia of the lungs in a high state of excitement, cramping fascia on veins which is bound to stop flow of blood to heart. No blood can pass through a vein that is closed by resistance, nor can it ever do it until resistance is suspended. Thus the cause of nerve irritation must be found and removed before the channels can relax and open sufficiently to admit the passage of the fluids being obstructed. And in order to remove this obstructing cause, we must go to the nerve supply of the lungs, or any other part of the body, and direct our attention to the cause of the nerve excitement, and that only; and prosecute the investigation to a finish. If the breathing be too fast and hurried, address your attention to the motor nerves, then to the sensory, for through them you regulate and reduce the excitement of the motor nerves of the arteries. As soon as sensation is reduced the motor and sensory circuit is completed and the labor of the artery is less, because of venous resistance having been removed. The circuit of electricity is complete as proven by the completed arterial and venous circuit for the reduction of motor irritation. The high temperature disappears because distress gives place to the normal, and recovery is the result.

CHAPTER X.

THE FASCIA.

Where Is Disease Sown?—An Illustration of Conception—The Greatest Problem—A Fountain of Supply—Fascia Omnipresent—Connection with Spinal Cord—Goes With and Covers All Muscles—Proofs in Contagion—Study of Nerves and Fascia—Tumefy—Tumefaction.

WHERE DISEASE IS SOWN.

Disease is evidently sown as atoms of gas fluids, or solids. A suitable place is necessary first to deposit the active principle of life, be that what it may. Then a responsive kind of nourishment must be obtained by the being to be developed. Thus we must find in animals that part of the body that can assist by action and by qualified food to develop the being in fœtal life. Reason calls the mind to the rule of man's gestative life first, and as a basis of thought, we look at the quickening atom, the coming being, when only by the aid of a powerful microscope can we see the vital germ. It looks like an atom of white fibrin or detached particle of fascia. It leaves one parent as an atom of fascia, and to live and grow, must dwell among friendly surroundings, and be fed by such food as contains albumen, fibrin and lymph; also the nerve generating power and qualities, as it then and there begins to construct a suitable form in which to live and flourish. And as the fascia is the best suited with nerves, blood, and white corpuscles, it is but reasonable to look for the part that is composed of the greatest per cent of fascia, and expect it, the germ, to dwell there for support and growth.

AN ILLUSTRATION OF CONCEPTION.

When you follow the germ from father until it has left his system of fascia, we find it flourishing in the womb, which organ is almost a complete being of itself. The center, origin, and mother of all fascias. It there dwells and grows to birth, and appears as a completed being, a product of the life giving powers of the fascia.

With this foundation established we think we prove conception, growth, and cause of all diseases to be in the fascia.

As this philosophy has chosen the fascia as a foundation on which to stand, we hope the reader will chain his patience for a few minutes on the subject of the fascia, and its relation to vitality. It stands before the philosopher as one of, if not the deepest living problems ever brought before the mind of man.

We will ask your attention in the attached effort to describe the fascia at greater length: It being that principle that sheathes, permeates, divides and sub-divides every portion of all animal bodies; surrounding and penetrating every muscle and all its fibers—every artery, and every fiber and principle thereunto belonging, and grows more wonderful as your eye is turned upon the venous system with its great company of lymphatics, which supplies the water of life, used to reduce too heavily thickened blood of the veins, as it approaches the heart on its journey, to be renewed after purification and thrown back into the arteries to patrol, nourish and supply from headquarters to the videts of this great moving army of life, the substance of which we are now speaking.

THE GREATEST PROBLEM.

The fascia is universal in man and equal in self to all other parts, and stands before the world to-day the greatest problem, the most pleasing thought. It carries to the mind of the philosopher the evidence, absolute, that it is the "material man," and the dwelling place his of spiritual being. It is the house of God, the dwelling place of the Infinite so far as man is concerned. It is the fort which the enemy of life takes by conquest through disease and winds up the combat and places thereon the black flag of "no quarters." That enemy is sure to capture all forts known as human beings at some time, although the engagement may last for many years. Procrastination of surrender can only be obtained by giving timely support to the supply of nourishment, with an unobstructed condition, kept up in favor of the nerves interested in the renewal of the human system, that powerful life force that is bequeathed to man and all other beings, and acts through the fascia of man and beast.

96

A FOUNTAIN OF SUPPLY.

The fascia gives one of, if not the greatest problems to solve as to the part it takes in life and death. It belts each muscle, vein, nerve, and all organs of the body. It is almost a network of nerves, cells and tubes, running to and from it; it is crossed and filled with, no doubt, millions of nerve centers and fibers to carry on the work of secreting and excreting fluid vital and destructive. By its action we live, and by its failure we shrink, or swell, and die. Each muscle plays its part in active life. Each fiber of all muscles owes its pliability to that yielding septum-washer, that gives all muscles help to glide over and around all adjacent muscles and ligaments, without friction or jar. It not only lubricates the fibers but gives nourishment to all parts of the body. Its nerves are so abundant that no atom of flesh fails to get nerve and fluid supply therefrom.

FASCIA OMNIPRESENT.

This life is surely too short to solve the uses of the fascia in animal forms. It penetrates even its own finest fibers to supply and assist its gliding elasticity. Just a thought of the completeness and universality in all parts, even though you turn the visions of your mind to follow the infinitely fine nerves. There you see the fascia, and in your wonder and surprise, you exclaim, "Omnipresent in man and all other living beings of the land and sea."

Other great questions come to haunt the mind with joy and admiration, and we can see all the beauties of life on exhibition by that great power with which the fascia is endowed. The soul of man with all the streams of pure living water seems to dwell in the fascia of his body.

Does it not throw hot shot and shells of thought into man's famishing chamber of reason; to feel that he has seen by thought the frame work of life the dwelling place on which life sojourns? He feels that he can find all disturbing causes of life, the place that diseases germinate and grow, the seeds of disease and death.

CONNECTION WITH THE SPINAL CORD.

As life finds its general nutrient law in the fascia and its nerves, we must connect them to the great source of supply by a cord running the length of the spine, by which all nerves are supplied by the brain. The cord throws out and supplies millions of nerves by which all organs and parts are supplied with the elements of motion, all go to and terminate in that great system, the fascia.

As we dip our cups deeper and deeper into the ocean of thought we feel that the solution of life and health is close to the field of the telescope of our mental search lights, and soon we will find the road to health so plainly written that the wayfaring man cannot err though he be a fool.

GOES WITH AND COVERS ALL MUSCLES.

As the student of anatomy explores the subject under his knife and microscope he easily finds this membrane goes with and covers all muscles, tendons and fibers, and separates them even to the least fiber. All organs have a covering of this substance, though they may have names to suit the organs, surfaces or parts spoken of.

We write much of the universality of the fascia to impress the reader with the idea that this connecting substance must be free at all parts to receive and discharge all fluids, if healthy to appropriate and use in sustaining animal life, and eject all impurities that health may not be impaired by the dead and poisoning fluids. Thus a knowledge of the universal extent of the fascia is almost imperative, and is one of the greatest aids to the person who seeks cause of disease. He of all men should know more of the fascia, and when disease is local or general. That the fascia and its nerves demand his attention first, and on his knowledge of the same, much of his success, and the life of his patients do depend.

Will the student of Osteopathy stop just a moment and see his medical cotemporary plow the skin with the needle of his hypodermic syringe. He drives it into and unloads his morphine and other poisonous drugs under the skin, and into the very center of the nerves of the superficial fascia. He produces paralysis of all nerves by this method, just as certainly as if he had put his poison in the cerebellum, but not so certain to produce instantaneous death as to unload in the brain. But if he is faithfully ignorant, he will kill just as certainly at one place as the other, because the poisonous effects can be easily taken to every fiber of the whole body by the nerves and fibers of the fascia.

When you deal with the fascia you deal and do business with the branch offices of the brain, and under the general corporation law, the same as the brain itself, and why not treat it with the same degree of respect?

The doctor of medicine does effectual work through the medium of the fascia. Why not you relax, contract, stimulate and clean the whole system of all diseases by that willing and sufficient power to renovate all parts of the system, from deadly compounds that generate through delay and stagnation of fluids while in the fascia.

Our school is young, but the laws that govern life are as old as the hours of all ages. We may find much that has never been written nor practiced before, but all such discoveries are truths born with the birth of eternity, old as God and as true as life.

The difference between a philosopher and a less powerful thinker is one observes alone, and depends on his own powers of mind to arrive at truth. Another lacks self confidence and mental energy.

PROOFS IN CONTAGION.

If disease is so highly attenuated, so etherial, and penetrable in quality, and multiple in atoms; and a breath of air two quarts or more taken into the lungs fully charged with contagion, how many thousand air cells could be impregnated by one single breath? Say we take a case of measles into a schoolroom of sixty pupils, in a warm and poorly oxygenized atmosphere all day, would not the living gas thrown off from active measles enter and irritate the air cells and close the most irritable cells with the poisonous gas retained for active development in those womb-like departments in the lungs.

Now you have the seeds in thousands of cells, which are as vital and well supplied by nerves and blood as the womb itself. Would not reason see the development of millions more of the vital beings who get their nourishment from the vitality found in the human fascia, which comes nearer to the surface in the lungs than in any part of the system, except it be the womb.

In proof of the certainty of measles being taken up by the lungs at one breath and caught by the secretions and conveyed to the universal system of fascia to develop the contagion, I will give the case of one of my boys who was sick with cold as I supposed; watering of eyes, cough, fever and headache. He was in the country about eight miles from home, and on our return stopped to get his books at a small school house. He ran in, picked up his books that were lying upon the desk, walked the length of the room which was about forty feet, was not there over one-half minute and in just nine days forty-two children broke out with measles. So certain is contagion to be taken up by the nerves and vitalizing fluids of the fascia.

It seems that all the fascia needs to develop anything is to have the seed planted in its arms for construction, the work will be done, labeled, and handed out for inspection by the inspectors of all works.

STUDY OF NERVES AND FASCIA.

We must remember as we reason on the power of life which is located in the fascia, that it occupies the whole body, and should we find a local region that is disordered and wish to, we can relieve that part through that local plexus of nerves which controls that organ and division. Thus your attention should be directed to all nerves of that part. Sensory, to modify sensation, blood must not be let run to the part by wild motion, its flow must be gentle to suit the demands of nutrition, otherwise weakness takes the place of strength, then we lose the benefits of the nerves of nutrition, by which strength of all systems of force are kept in action during life.

Suppose the nerves that supply the lungs with motion should stop, the lungs would stop also; suppose they should half stop, the lungs would surely half stop. Now we must reason, if we succeed in relieving lungs, that all kinds of nerves are found in them. The lungs move, thus you find motor; they have feeling, thus the sensory; they grow by nutrition, (thus the nutrient nerves;) they move by will, or without it; they have a voluntary and involuntary system; they move in sleep by the involuntary system.

The blood supply comes under the motor system of nerves, and delivers at proper places for the convenience of the nerves of nutrition. The sensory nerves limit the supply of arterial blood to the quantity necessary, as the construction is going on by each successive stroke of the heart. They limit the action of the lungs, receive and expel air in quantities sufficient to keep up purity of the blood, etc. With this foundation we observe if too great action of the motor nerves, shows by breathing too often to be normal, we are admonished to reduce breathing by addressing attention to the sensory nerves of lungs, in order that the blood may pass through the veins, whose irritability has refused to receive the blood, farther than arterial terminals. So soon as sensation is reduced relaxation of nerve fibers of veins tolerates the passage of venous blood, which is deposited in the spongy portions of the lungs in such quantities as to overcome the activity of the nerves of renovation that accompanies the fascia in its process of ejection of all fluids that have been detained an abnormal time, first in the region of the fascia, then in the arterial and venous circulation. Thus you see what must be done. The veins as channels must carry away all blood as soon as it has deposited its nutrient supplies to the places for which it is constructed, otherwise, by delay vitality by asphyxia is lost to the blood which calls a greater force of the arterial pumps to drive the blood through the parts, ruptures its capillaries and deposits the blood in the mucous membrane; until nerves of the fascia becomes powerless by surrounding pressure, which causes through the sensory nerves an irritability at the heart, which puts in force all its powers of motion.

TUMEFY, TUMEFACTION.

Webster's definition of tumefaction is to swell by any fluids or solids being detained abnormally at any place in the body.

The location may be in, or on any part of the system. No part is exempt; even the brain, heart, lungs, liver, stomach and bowels, bladder, kidneys, uterus, lymphatics, glands, nerves, veins, arteries, skin and all membranes are subject to swellings locally or generally, and with equal certainty they perish and shrink away. If either condition should exist death to the parts or all of the body will occur from want of nutrition. Instance, in lung fever which begins when swelling is established in lymphatics of lungs, trachea, nostrils, throat and face. At once you see the pressure on the nerve fibers compressed to such degree that they cannot operate excretories of lungs or any part of the pulmonary, system. Veins, suspended by irritation of the nerves, arteries are excited to fever heat in action with increase of tumefaction. A tumefying condition undoubtedly marks the beginning of all catarrhal diseases. Its ravages extend to the diseases of the fall and winter seasons. They are so marked on examination that the most skeptical cannot dispute or doubt the truth of this position. In fact he is already committed to a belief that there is something in the fluids that he must purify by the chemical process of drugs.

MEDICAL DOCTOR'S TREATMENT.

He looks on, and treats winter diseases with powerful purgatives, sweats, blisters, hot and cold applications with a view to remove congesting fluids. He is not very certain which team of medical power he can depend on. He hitches up many kinds of drugs hoping that a few of them may be able to carry the burden. He bridles his horses with opium, loads them down with purgative powders, and whips them through with castor oil, and for fear they will not travel fast enough he uses as a spur a delicately formed instrument known as the hypodermic syringe. He punches and prods until his horses fall exhausted. Disease and death should give him a large pension for the assistance he has rendered in their service. All is guess work whose father and mother are "Tradition and Ignorance." Ignorance of the kind that is wholly inexcusable to anyone but a medical doctor. An Osteopath who does not understand the general law of tumefaction of the whole system is not excusable from the fact that tumefaction, disease and death are so plainly written on the face of all diseases that the blind need not have eyes to see, nor the philosopher any brain to enable him to know this foundation is the highest known truth of all man's intellectual possessions. Thus by the law of tumefaction, death can and does succumb to its indomitable will. Observations without record will show any fair minded person that tumefaction does cause death in the majority of cases. But another power is equally as effective in destruction of life which is just the reverse of tumefaction. It destroys by withholding nutrition and all of the fluids; the effect is starvation, shrinkage and death. Thus you see it is equally certain in results. In the one case death ensues from an overplus of unappropriated fluids of nutrition, in the other there is no appropriation to sustain animal life and the patient dies from starvation. The same law holds good in the parts as well as in the whole body.

CHAPTER XI.

FEVERS.

Be Armed With Facts—Union of Human Gases With Oxygen—Fever
and Nettle-rash. Nature Constructs for a Wise Purpose—Processes of
Life Must be Kept in Motion—No Satisfaction from Authors—
Animal Heat—Semeiology—Symptomatology—Definition of
Fever—Fevers only ⊕ts—Result of Stoppages of Vein or Artery—
Aneurisms.

BE ARMED WITH FACTS.

When we reason for causes we must begin with facts, and hold them
constantly in line for action, and use, all the time. It would be good
advice never to enter a contest without your saber is of the purest
steel of reason. By such only can you cut your way to the magazine
of truth.

As we line up to learn something of the cause of fever, we are met by
heat, a living fact. Does that put the machinery of your mind in
motion? If not, what will arouse your mental energy? You see that
heat is not like cold. It is not a horse with eyes, head, neck, body,
limbs and tail; but it is as much of a being as the horse; it is a being of
heat. If cause made the horse, and cause made the heat, why not
devote all energy in seeking for cause in all disturbances of life?

UNION OF HUMAN GASES WITH OXYGEN.

Who says heat is not a union of the human gases with oxygen and
other substances as they pass out of the excretory system. By what
force do parts of the engine of life move? If by the motor power of
electricity, how fast must the heart or life current run to ignite the
gasolene of the body and set a person on fire and burn to fever heat?

If we know anything of the laws of electricity, we must know
velocity modulates its temperature. Thus heat and cold are the effect.

If we understand anatomy as we should, we know man is the greatest engine ever produced, complete in form, an electro-magnet, a motor, and would be incomplete if it could not burn its own gases.

When man, is said to have fever, he is only on "fire," to burn out the deadly gases, which a perverted, dirty, abnormal, laboratory, has allowed to accumulate by friction of the journals of his body, or in the supply of vital fluids. We are only complete when normal in all parts, —a true compass points to the normal only.

When reasoning on the fever subject would it not be strictly in line to suppose that the lowest perceptible grade of fever requires a less additional physical energy to remove some foreign body from the person, that at first would naturally show a very light effect upon the human system, which would be the effect of itchy sensation.

FEVER AND NETTLE-RASH.

Let us stop and reason. Might this effect (itching) not come from obstructed gases that flow through and from the skin? If gas should be detained in the system by the excretory ducts the substance closing the porous system would cause irritation of nerves, and increase the heart's action to such degree that the temperature is raised to fever heat, by the velocity with which electricity is brought into action. Electricity being the force that is naturally required to contract muscles and force gases from the body.

Let us advance higher in the scale of foreign bodies until we arrive to the condition of steam, which is more dense than gas. Would it not take more force to discharge it? By the same rule of reasoning we find water to be much thicker as an element than either gas or steam.

Then we have lymph as another element, albumen, fibrin, with all the elements found in arterial and venous blood, all of which forces required to circulate, pass through and out of the system, must be increased to suit. Therefore we are brought to this conclusion, that the different degrees of temperature do mark the density of the fluids with which the motor engine has to contend.

If gas produces an itching sensation, would it not be reasonable to suppose that the consistence of lymph would cause elevations on the skin, such as nettle-rash.

If this method of reasoning sustains us thus far, why not argue that albumen obstructed while in the system of the fascia would require a much greater force to put it through the skin. The excretions of the body would cause a much greater heat to even throw the albumen as far as the cuticle.

If a greater, with a greater velocity, why not grant to this as cause of the disturbance of motor energy equal to measles. Let us add to this albumen a quantity of fibrin, have we not cause to expect the energy hereby required to be equal to that nerve and blood energy found in smallpox?

If this be true, have we not a foundation in truth on which to base our conclusions? That the difference in forces manifested is the resistance offered by the difference in the consistence of devitalized fluids which the nerves and fibers of the fascia labor to excrete.

NATURE CONSTRUCTS TO SUIT A WISE PURPOSE.

By close observation the philosopher who is hunting to acquaint himself with the laws of cause and effect, finds upon his voyages as an explorer, that nature as cause does construct for wise purposes; and shows as much wisdom in the construction and preparation of all bodies, beings and worlds, as the workings of those beings show when in action.

As life, the highest known principle sent forth by nature to vivify, construct and govern all beings, it is expected to be the indweller and operator, and one of the greatest perceivable and universal laws of nature. And when it becomes necessary to break the friendly relation between life and matter, nature closes up the channels of supply.

It may begin its work near the heart, at the origin of the greatest blood vessels, or do its work at any point. It may begin its closing process at the extremities of the veins or anywhere where exhausted vital fluids may enter for return to the heart for renewal by union with new material.

As nature is never satisfied with incompleteness in anything, all interferences from whatsoever cause are sufficient for nature to call a halt and begin the work of excavation by bringing the necessary fluids, already prepared in the chemical laboratory, to dissolve and wash away all obstructing deposits previous to beginning the work of reconstruction, which is to repair all injured parts of the machinery if disabled by atmospheric cause, poisons, or otherwise.

When nature renovates it is never satisfied to leave any obstruction in any part of the body. All the powers of its battery force are brought in line to do duty, and never stop short of completeness which ends in perfection.

All seasons of the year come and go, and we see year in and out the perpetual processes of construction of one class of bodies, and the passing away of others.

Vegetation builds forests, and cold builds mountains of ice to be dissolved and sent into the ocean to purify the water, and keep the brines from drying to powder, as salt.

PROCESSES OF LIFE MUST BE KEPT IN MOTION.

All the processes of earth-life, must be kept in perpetual motion to cultivate and be kept in healthy condition, or the world would wither and die, and go to the tombs of space, to join the funeral procession of other dead worlds. Thus you see all nature comes and goes by the fiat of wisely adjusted laws.

NO SATISFACTION FROM AUTHORS.

Read all the authors from Æsculapius to this date, and all combined leave the inquirers without a single fact as to the cause or causes of fever.

One says fever may come from too much carbon. Another says chemical defects may be the cause.

I would like to agree with some of the good men of our date or the ancient theorists if I could, but they, both dead and alive, are a blank except the tons of paper they have covered all over with conjectures, and closed out by the words "Perhaps so's and howevers" spoken in all tongues and languages on earth.

All have explored for centuries for the cause of fevers, and on return from their multiple voyages say, we hope some day to find the cause. We have killed many dogs experimenting, but have failed to find the cause of fever.

ANIMAL HEAT.

To think of fever, we think of animal heat. By habit we want to know how great the heat is. We measure by a yard stick till we find we have 100°, 102°, 104°, to 106°, at this point we stop as we find too many yards of red calico to suit the size of the purse of life. Which we think cannot consume more than 106 yards of heat. We begin to ask for the substances that are more powerful than fire. We try all known fire compounds and fail. The fire department had done faithful work, and all it could bring to bear on the fire. It had put on hose and steam, knocked shingles off and windows out, but not until the fire had ruined the house with all its inside and outside usefulness and beauties. Another and another house gets on fire and burns just as the first did. All are content to see the ruins and say it is the will of the Lord; never thinking for a moment that it was with the aid of the heart that the brain burned up the body.

Of what use is a knowledge of anatomy to man if he overlooks cause and effect in the results obtained by the machinery that anatomy should teach? He finds each part connected to all others with the wisdom that has given a set of plans and specifications that are without a flaw or omission. The body generates its own heat and modulates to suit climate and season. It can generate through its electro-motor system far beyond the kindly normal, to the highest known fever heat, and is capable of modulations far above or below normal. A knowledge of Osteopathy will prepare you to bring the system under the rulings of the physical laws of life. Fever is electric heat only.

SEMEIOLOGY.

(Med.) The science of the signs or symptoms of disease.

SYMPTOMATOLOGY.

The doctrine of symptoms; that part of the science of medicine which treats of the symptoms of disease. Semeiology.

These definitions are from Webster's International Dictionary, considered by all English speaking people as a standard authority. Both words are chosen names to represent that system of guess work, which is now and has been used as a method of ascertaining what disease is or might be. It is supposed to be the best method known to date to classify or name diseases, after which guessing begins in earnest. What kinds of poisons, how much and how often to use them, and guess how much good or how much harm is being done to the sick person.

To illustrate more forcibly, to the mind of the reader that such system though honored by age is only worthy the name of guess work, as shown by the following standard authority on fevers:

POTTER'S DEFINITION OF FEVER.

"Fever is a condition in which there are present the phenomena of rise of temperature, quickened circulation, marked tissue change, and disordered secretions.

"The primary cause of the fever phenomena is still a mooted (discussed and debated) question, and is either a disorder of the sympathetic nervous system giving rise to disturbances of the vaso-motor filaments, or a derangement of the nerve centers located adjacent to the corpus striatum, which have been found, by experiment, to govern the processes of heat production, distribution, and dissipation.

"Rise of temperature is the pre-eminent feature of all fevers, and can only be positively determined by the use of the clinical thermometer. The term feverishness is used when the temperature ranges from 99°

to 100° fahr.; slight fever if 100° or 101°; moderate, 102° or 103°; high if 104° or 105° and intense if it exceed the latter. The term hyperpyrexia is used when the temperature shows a tendency to remain at 106° fahr. and above.

"Quickened circulation is the rule in fevers, the frequency usually maintaining a fair ratio with the increase of the temperature. A rise of one degree fahr. is usually attended with an increase of eight to ten beats of the pulse per minute.

"The following table gives a fair comparison between temperature and pulse:—

TABLE OF DEGREES.

A temperature of					
	98° corresponds	to a	pulse of		60°
"	99°	"	"	"	70°
"	100°F	"	"	"	80°
"	101°F	"	"	"	90°
"	102°F	"	"	"	100°
"	103°F	"	"	"	110°
"	104°F	"	"	"	120°
"	105°F	"	"	"	130°
"	106°F	"	"	"	140°

"The tissue waste is marked in proportion to the severity and duration of the febrile phenomena, being slight or (nil) in febricula, and excessive in typhoid fever.

"The disordered secretions are manifested by the deficiency in the salivary, gastric, intestinal, and nephritic secretions, the tongue being furred, the mouth clammy, and there occurring anorexia, thirst, constipation, and scanty, high-colored acid urine."[6]

FEVERS ONLY EFFECTS.

Fevers are effects only. The cause may be far from mental conclusions. If we have a house with one bell, and ten wires each fastened to a door running to the center, all having wire connection and so arranged that to pull any one wire will set the bell in motion, and without an indicator you cannot tell which wire is disturbed, producing the effect or ringing of the bell at the center. An electrician would know at once the cause, but to discriminate and locate the wire disturbed is the study.

Before a bell can be heard from any door, the general battery must be charged. Thus you see but one source of supply. To better illustrate—we will take a house with eight rooms, and all supplied by one battery—one is a reception room, one a parlor, one a sitting room, one bed room, one cloak room, one dining room, one a kitchen, and one a basement room, all having wires and bells running to one bell in the clerk's office, which has an indicator for each room by numbers on its face. If the machinery is in good order he can call and answer correctly all the time and never make a mistake. But should he ring to call the cook and her bell keep on ringing and she and clerk could not stop it, and they summon an electrician, what would you think if he began at the parlor bell to adjust a trouble of the kitchen bell? Surely you would not have him treat the parlor bell first, because you know the cook could only answer by the effect, or rattling of the office bell. Hers is cause, sound at office, effect. Now to apply this illustration, we will say a system of bells and connecting wires run to all parts or rooms of the body, from the battery of power or the brain, conveyed by the strings of wires or nerves, that are put up and run to all active or vital parts of the body. Thus arranged we see how blood is driven to any part of the system, by the power that is sent over the nerves from the brain to the spinal cord, and from there to all nerves of each and all divisions of the body. Then your blood that has done its work in constructing parts or all of the system, entering veins to be returned to the heart for renewal. Each vein, great and small, has nerves with them as servants of power, to force blood back to heart through the different sets of tubes known as veins, and made to suit the duties they have to perform in the process of life. As it travels to the heart

111

with blood too thick to suit the lungs, the great system of lymphatics pour in water to suit demands, preparatory to entering the lungs to be purified and renewed. Thus you see nature has amply prepared all the machinery and power to prepare material and construct all parts, and when in normal condition the mind and wisdom of God is satisfied that the machine will go on and build and run according to the plan and specification. If this be true as nature proves at every point and principle, what can man do farther than plumb, line up, and trust to nature to get results desired, "life and health?" Can we add or suggest any improvement? If not, what is left for us to do is to keep bells, batteries and wires in normal place and trust to normal law as given by nature.

RESULT OF STOPPAGE OF VEIN OR ARTERY.

But few questions remain to be asked by the philosophical navigator when he sets sail to go to the cause of flux. Would he go to blood supply? Certainly, there must be supply previous to deposit. Reason would cause us to combine the fact that blood must be in perpetual motion from and to the heart during life, and that law is the fiat of all nature which is indispensable and absolute. Blood must not stop its motion nor be allowed to unduly deposit, as the heart's action is perpetual in motion. The work is complete of the heart if it delivers blood into the exploring arteries. Each division must to do its part fully as a normal heart does, or can in the greatest measure of health; and a normally formed heart is just as much interested in the blood that is running constantly for repairs and additions, as the whole system is on the arteries for supply. Thus you must have perfection in shape first, and from it to all parts as far as an artery reaches. All hindrances must be kept away from the arteries great and small. Health permits of no stopping of blood in either the vein or artery. If an artery cannot unload its consents a strain follows, and as an artery must have room to deposit its supplies it proceeds to build other vessels adjacent to the points of obstruction.

ANEURISMS.

Some are builded to enormous sizes. We call them aneurisms or accommodation chambers, builded by nature's constructing ability of the arteries as deposits for blood. The artery should pass farther on, thus you by reason must know an obstruction has limited the flow of blood, and the tumor is only an effect, and obstruction is the cause of all abnormal deposits, either from vein or artery. Unobstructed blood cannot form a tumor, nor allow inharmony to dwell in any part of the system. Flux is an effect, blood supply and circulation both at variation from normal. An artery finds veins of bowels irritated and contracted to such degree that arterial blood cannot enter veins with cargo of blood at all, and deposits its blood at terminal points in mucous membrane of bowels, and when membrane fails to hold all blood so delivered, then the first blood which dies of asphyxia finds an outlet into the bowels to be carried off and out by peristaltic actions. Thus you have a continuous deposit and discharge for arterial blood until death stops the supply.

CHAPTER XII.

SCARLET FEVER AND SMALLPOX.

As defined by Allopathy—Scarlet Fever as Defined by Osteopathy—Smallpox—Power to Drive Greater Than in Measles.

AS DEFINED BY ALLOPATHY.

"Scarlet fever begins with a short period of tired feeling. A short period of chilly sensation, fullness of eyes and sore throat. In a few hours fever begins with great heat of back of head. It soon extends all over the body, sick stomach and vomiting generally accompany the disease. Rash of a red color beginning on back, and extends to throat and limbs. About the second or third day, the fever is very high, from 100° to 104° and generally lasts to fifth and seventh day, at which time fever begins to diminish, with itching over the body. The skin at this time throws off all of the dead scales that had been red rash in the fore-part of the disease. Often the lining membranes of the mouth, throat and tonsils slough and bleed. Also pus is often formed just under the skin in front of the throat. Such cases usually die.[7]

ALLOPATHY."

SCARLET FEVER AS DEFINED BY OSTEOPATHY.

Is a disease generally of the early spring and late fall seasons. Generally comes with cold and damp weathers during east winds. It begins with sore throat, chilly and tired feelings, followed with headache and vomiting. In a few hours chilly feeling leaves and fever sets in very high, burns your hands. The patient is rounded in chest, abdomen, face and limbs by congestion of the fascia and all of the lymphatic glands. This stagnation will soon begin its work of fermentation of the fluids of fascia, then you see the rash. If you do not want to see the rash and sloughing of throat, with a dead patient,

I would advise you to train your guns on the blood, nerves, and lymphatics of the fascia and stop the cause at once, or quit.

OSTEOPATHY.

SMALLPOX.

If we give a thought to the action of the electro-motor force, we would be constrained to believe that a power that could drive gas through a body of great density, would be much less than one that could force lymph through the same density. The same of albumen.

POWER TO DRIVE GREATER THAN IN MEASLES.

Thus in smallpox the motor energy must be equal to the force that would convey albumen through all tissues. Measles would be less, and so on according to the thickness of the fluids present. Thus you see the power to drive dead fluids from fascia must be much greater in smallpox than in cases of measles. Then we must see why the pulse of smallpox is so powerful during development of the pox. After killing the fluids by retention in the fascia of the skin, a greater force yet is created by hurting nerve fibers of fascia; then the motor energy appears and all the powers of life go to help the arteries force fluids through the skin and push to and leave them in the fascia of the skin to be eliminated as best it can. In some parts elimination fails, such places are called pox. They supurate and drop out leaving a pit (the pox mark). Now had the nerves of the skin and fascia not been irritated to contract the skin against the fascia passing its dead fluids through the excretory ducts of the skin, we probably would have no eruption. It is not quite reasonable to conclude that after the heart overloads the fascia and the nerves lose their control by pressure of fluids, that all that is left is chemical action to the production of pus, which throws it out of fascia in intervening spaces? Then should the fascia have greater death of its substances, we have one spot to run into others, and we have "confluent smallpox."

CHAPTER XIII.

A CHAPTER OF WONDERS AND SOME VALUABLE QUESTIONS.

Wonders on the Increase—What Is Life?—How Is Action
Produced—Acquaint Yourself With the Machinery—Duty of the
Osteopath—Formation of Sacrum—The Pelvis—Appearance of
Œdema—Do All Diseases Have Appearance in Œdema.

WONDERS ON THE INCREASE.

Wonders are daily callers, and seem greatly on the increase during
the Eighteenth century. As we read history we learn that no one
hundred years of the past has produced wonders in such number
and variety. Stupid systems of government have given place to
better and wiser. Voyages of the ocean have had months by sail
reduced to days by steam. Journeys over land that would require six
months by horse and ox, are now accomplished in six days by rail.
Our law, medical and other schools of five and seven years, are now
but two or three; and the graduates of such schools are far superior
in useful knowledge to those of the five and seven. And no wonder
at that, for the facilities for giving the pupil an education are so far
superior that the knowledge sought, can be obtained in less time.
Our schools are not intended to use the greatest number of days that
are allotted to man. But at this day schooling and learning mean, to
obtain useful knowledge in the quickest way that a thoroughness can
be obtained. If there is any method by which arithmetic can be
taught so as to master it in thirty days instead of thirty months let us
have it. We want knowledge, we are willing to pay for it, we want all
we pay for, and we want our heads kept out of the sausage-mill of
time wasting.

A great question now stands before us: What are the possibilities of
mind to improve our methods of gaining knowledge, shorten time,
and getting greater and better results? I am free to say the question is
too momentous to form an answer, as each day brings a new
wonder, to the man or woman who reasons on cause, and gives
demonstrations by effects.

WHAT IS LIFE?

The philosopher who first asked that question no one knows. But all intelligent persons are interested in the solution of this problem, at least to know some tangible reason why it is called life; whether life is personal or so arranged that it might be called an individualized principle of nature.

I wish to think for a time on this line, because we should make a wise handling of the machinery of the body.

If life in man has been formed to suit the size and duties of the being; if life has a living and separate personage, then we should be governed by such reasons as would give it the greatest chance to go on with its labors in the bodies of man and beast.

We know by experience that a spark of fire will start the principles of powder into motion, which, were it not stimulated by the positive principle of father nature, which finds this germ lying quietly in the womb of space, would be silently inactive for all ages, without being able to move or help itself, save for the motor principle of life given by the father of all motion.

HOW IS ACTION PRODUCED.

Right here we could and should ask the question: Is this action produced by electricity put in motion, or is it the active principle that comes as a spiritual man? If so, it is useless to try, or hope to know what life is in its minutia. But we do know that life can only display its natural forces by the visible action of the forms it produces.

If we inspect man as a machine, we find a complete building, a machine that courts inspection and criticism. It demands a full exploration of all its parts with their uses. Then the mind is asked to see or find the connection between the physical, and the spiritual. By nature you can reason on the roads that the powers of life are arranged to suit its system of motion.

If life is an individualized personage, as we might express that mysterious something, and it must have definite arrangements by which it can be united and act with matter; then we are admonished to acquaint ourselves with the arrangements of those natural connections, the one or many, as they are connected to all parts of the completed being.

As motion is the first and only evidence of life, by this thought we are conducted to the machinery through which life works to accomplish these results.

ACQUAINT YOURSELF WITH THE MACHINERY.

If the brain be that division in which force is generated or stored, you must at all hazards acquaint yourself with that structure of this machine; trace the connection from brain to heart, from heart to lungs, and other organs that can be acted upon by the brain, whose duty may be to construct the fleshy and bony parts of the body. Trace from the brain to the chemical laboratories, and note their action as they unite and prepare blood and other fluids, that are used in the economy of this vital, self-constructing and self-moving wonder, commonly known as man; wherein life and matter do unite, and express their friendly relation one with the other; and while this relation exists we have the living man only, expressing and proving the relation that can exist between life and matter, from the lowest living atom, to the greatest worlds. They can only express form and action by this law. Harmony only dwells where obstructions do not exist.

DUTY OF THE OSTEOPATH.

The Osteopath finds here the field in which he can dwell forever. His duties as a philosopher admonish him, that life and matter can be united, and that union cannot continue with any hindrance to the free and absolute motion. Therefore his duty is to keep away from the track all that will hinder the complete passage of the forces of the nervous system, that by that power the blood may be delivered and adjusted, to keep the system in normal condition. Here is your duty; do it well, if you wish to succeed.

FORMATION OF SACRUM.

We believe only when we do not know. Belief and doubt are equal terms. If we believe the sacrum is formed by a local system, then we can or will have cause to believe that the rectum and colon appear after the outer skin is in process of forming. For want of the truths we are left in speculative doubt. I believe the lower bowels are formed by local machinery that receives and appropriates to the purpose of construction of such parts or organs as nature designs to be used there. If we dissect a chicken as soon as hatched we will find the colon beginning at rectum and complete in form, but not connected to the small intestines.

THE PELVIS.

To get more directly at the point I want to make I will say I have some reasons to believe that the lower bowels are builded from rectum to the vermiform appendix, by acts of pelvis. It may be well to state that I have seen formation of rectum and colon in the chicken, before the small intestines were visible at all. Then in same chicken I saw, liver, lung, crop and gizzard, and only one artery in the region of the small intestines. From this I was led to believe that the pelvis did much of the forming of the viscera. If so, then we could look for much relief through the system of the pelvis.

APPEARANCE OF ŒDEMA.

Œdema is the one word that appears to be at the first showing of life and death in animal forms. Previous to death by general swelling of system, a watery swelling of fascia and lymphatics, even to those of nerve fibers. If a disease should destroy life by withholding all fluids, we can trace such cause in the beginning to a time when there was watery swelling of the centers of nerves of nutrition, to such amount as to cut off nerve supply until sensation ceased to renovate and keep off accumulating fluids so long that fermentation did the work of heating till all fluids had dried up, and the channels of supply closed by adhesive inflammation, and death follows by the law of general atrophy.

DO ALL DISEASES HAVE BEGINNING IN ŒDEMA?

To assert that all diseases have their beginning in œdema may be wide in range, but we often find one principle to rule over much territory. "Instance:" Mind is the supreme ruler of all beings, from the mites of life to the monsters of the land and sea. Thus we see a ruling principle is without limit. The same of numbers. By heat all metals melt to fluidity; acids must have oxygen to begin as solvents in most metals. We only speak imperfectly of some common laws to prepare the student to think on the line of probabilities as I hold them out for consideration. Suppose we begin at the atoms of fluids such as enter to construct animal or vegetable forms, and pen up till decomposition begins. By such delay does not nature call a halt and refuse to obey the laws of construction and let all other supplies pile up even to death? Is not all this the result of œdema? Œdema surely begins with the first tardy atom of matter.

Pneumonia begins by its œdematous accumulations of dead atoms, even to the death of the whole body, all having found a start in atoms only.

QUESTIONS FOR THE OSTEOPATH.

We will close this chapter by propounding a few questions which the Osteopath should keep in mind.

Are the human and animal forms complete as working machines?

Has nature furnished man with powers to make his bones; give them the needed shapes of durable material, strong in kind?

Does a section in nature's law provide fastenings to hold these to one another?

Then another question arises: How will this body move, and where and how is the force applied?

Where and how is this force obtained?

How is it generated and supplied to these parts of motion?

What makes these muscles, ligaments, nerves, veins, arteries?

Are they self-forming, or has nature prepared machinery to make them?

Does animal life contain knowledge and force to construct all of the parts of man?

Can it run the machine after it has finished it?

By what power does it move?

Is there a blood vessel running to all parts of this body to supply all these demands?

If it has a battery of force, where is it?

What does it use for force?

Is it electricity? If so how does it collect and use this substance?

How does it convey its powers to any or all places?

How does the man keep warm without fire?

How does he build and lose flesh all the time?

Where and how is the supply made and delivered to proper places?

How is it applied and what holds it to its place when adjusted?

What makes it build the house of life?

Do demand and supply govern the work? If not, what does?

Are the laws of animal life sufficient to do all this work of building and repairing wastes and keep it in running condition?

If it does, what can man do or suggest to help it?

Is this machine capable of being run fast or slow if need be?

Does man have in him some kind of chemical laboratory that can turn out such products as he needs to fill all his physical demands?

If by heat, exercise, or any other cause he gets warm, can that chemistry cool him to normal?

If too cold can it warm him? Can it adjust him to heat and cold?

If so, how is it done? Is the law of life and longevity fully vindicated in man's make up?

CHAPTER XIV.

Has Man Degenerated?

The Advent of Man—Care of the Stock Raiser—Mental Degeneration Makes It Unpleasant for an Original Thinker—Original Thinkers of the Ancients—Methods of Healing—Failure of Allopathy—Primitive Man—Evidences of Prehistoric Man—Mental Dwarfage.

THE ADVENT OF MAN.

The exact time when man's foot appeared on the earth, no record shows. A knowledge of his advent might be profitable. The unwritten history of the human races with the genius or lack of genius, might to us be an open book of knowledge. As it is not supposable that the mind of man has just become observingly active in the last few centuries, absolute evidence of purer and deeper reason than we have been able to present, stand recorded on the faces of many valuable "lost arts" which we have never been able to equal. Is it not very reasonable to suppose that the powers of mind have wonderfully degenerated from some cause?

CARE OF THE STOCK RAISER.

The stock raiser carefully preserves the best and most healthy of the males and females of his flocks and herds for breeding purposes, that their offspring might be healthy and well developed, for the purposes for which he raises them. As a result he raises stock from the poultry house up, with marked improvement in form, strength and usefulness. Should he be foolish enough to kill off all the healthy and well developed males as they appear in his herds of cattle and other stock, for one or two centuries, would any one with average intelligence suppose that the standard of animals would or could be kept up, by breeding from the unfortunate stock, that had been pierced through the lungs while fighting with more powerful animals. If for breeding purposes he would save calves, colts, lambs, pigs, goats or any other young males to breed from, that had had a leg frozen off, one or both eyes plucked out, necks and ears torn by panthers, what would you think of the man's sanity?

On this line we would ask what has been the procedure of all nations? Has it not been to select the strong and healthy males, drive them out to the field of battle, destroy a million or more of the strongest men, as our war of the sixties shows. Since that war closed the fathers of our children are mainly the crippled, worn out, and degenerated physical wrecks, with the assistance of the refused, who for lack of physical ability were barred from entering the United States' service. Such physical and mental wrecks are the fathers of the children born during the last thirty years. Every healthy young lady who married and became a mother after the early sixties, had to select a husband from a war or hereditary wreck. From that degenerated stock of human beings our asylums are filled, and the beams of the gallows pulled down by the weight of the bodies of those mental dwarfs. Run this train of reason back for a few hundred or thousand of years,—this degenerating force, bearing upon the offspring, and is it a wonder that we have physical and mental wrecks all over the country?

MENTAL DEGENERATION MAKES IT UNPLEASANT FOR THE ORIGINAL THINKER.

Now if we have been mentally degenerating, killing our best men back for a few thousand years time, and still have a few left who are fairly good reasoners, what was their mental powers then, compared with now? They could think from native ability; we only through acquired ability by our methods of education. Should an original thinker occasionally appear from the crippled and maimed, he will have much that is unpleasant to contend with, unless he is generous enough to credit the cause to an effect produced by the lack of mental and physical forces in the sires just described. A man or woman who is able to reason, cannot afford to wear out his or her physical and mental forces by spending time in tiresome discussions with such blank masses, who are very fortunate to have intelligence enough to make a living under the methods that require the least mental action.

It would not be manly nor lady like to allow a feeling of combattiveness to arise and spend your forces on such persons. Prenatal causes have dropped them where they are, and a philosopher knows he must submit to the conditions, and he is sorrowful in place of vengeful and vindicative, and all that is left for him to do is to trim his lamps and let the lights defend themselves.

ORIGINAL THINKERS OF THE ANCIENTS.

On this line we have much to think of. Anciently they did think: Great minds existed then, as is evidenced by the architecture displayed in constructing temples and pyramids. As in philosophy, chemistry, and mathematics, they stand to-day as living facts of their intelligence. In some ways we are equal and even surpass the ancients. Before the establishment of religious and political governments, national and tribal creeds, to sustain which the powerful minds and bodies of thousands and millions have been slain and their wise councils prohibited by death. Reason says under the circumstances we must kindly make and do the best we can in our day and time. No doubt their religion was better than ours, before they began to fight about their gods and governments.

METHODS OF HEALING.

Some evidence crops out now and then that their methods of healing were natural and wisely applied, and crowned with good results. As far as history speaks of the ancient healing arts they were logical, philosophical, good in results and harmless. It is true enough that we have great systems of chemistry that are useful in the mechanical arts, but very limited in their uses in the healing arts. In fact, a very great per cent of the gray-haired philosophers of all medical schools, unhesitatingly assert that the world would be better off without them. These conclusions are sent forth by competent and honest investigators, who have tested all known methods and medicines, and carefully observed the results from a quarter to a half a century. Let us call it "a trade," as the use of drugs is not a science.

The author will now say, the health hunter in a majority of cases, when he administers drugs, gives one dose for health and nine for the dollar.

As it becomes necessary to throw off oppressive governments, it becomes just as necessary to throw off other useless customs, without which no substitute has ever been received.

FAILURE OF ALLOPATHY.

Allopathy, a school of medicine known and fostered by all nations, drove on with its exploring teams; gave up the search, went into camp and builded temples to the god who purged, puked, perspired, opiated, drank whiskey and other stimulants; destroyed its thousands, ruined nations, established whiskey saloons, opium dens, insane asylums, naked mothers and hungry babies, and still cries aloud, and says: "Come unto me and I will give you rest. I have opium, morphine, and whiskey by the barrel. I am the god of all healing knowledge, and want to be so recognized by people and statute. I do not wish to be annoyed by Eclecticism, Homœopathy, Christian science, massage, Swedish movements, nor Osteopathy. I do not like Osteopathy any better than I do a tiger. It scratches me and tears away all my disciples. I cannot destroy it. It uses neither opium nor whiskey, and it is impossible to catch it asleep. It scratches us, and has scratched our power out of four states during the last twelve months, with no telling where it will scratch next time. We must prepare for more war, I have heard from my scouts that on its flag the inscription reads thus: 'No quarters for allopathy in particular and none at all for any schools of medicine farther than surgery, and war to the hilt on three-fourths of that as practiced in the present day. The use of the knife in everything and for everything must be stopped; not by statute law, but through a higher education of the masses, which will give them more confidence in nature's ability to heal.'"

PRIMITIVE MAN.

It is reasonable to suppose that the mind that constructed man was fully competent to undertake and complete the being to suit the purpose for which he was designed. After giving him physical perfection in every limb, organ, or part of his body, it is reasonable to suppose, that at that time, he gave him all the mental powers needed for all purposes during the life of his race, and with that perfection in the physical, it is supposable he approached very nearly to intellectual perfection. He was a mathematician, not by collegiate process, but by native ability. He did not have to take a course in a university to study chemistry, because of the fact that he was a chemist when he was born. Possibly he could speak or understand all languages spoken by the human tongue, from the powers of his mind, which occupied a pure and healthy physique. In a word he was well made and fully endowed with all the physical and mental forces necessary to the whole journey of his life. Now a question arises: "When did he begin to degenerate physically and mentally?" Let us reason some on this line, which seems to be a rather solid foundation, and as history is young itself, and has imperfectly recorded only such events as have transpired during a few centuries, with records imperfectly preserved.

EVIDENCES OF PREHISTORIC MAN.

We see evidences all along the journey of prehistoric man's life, though the being and his bones have been mostly obliterated; we see close to his bony remains the stone axe, the flint-dart. We find acres of ground in many places close to mounds and caves, with countless millions of slivers that have been scaled from flints and formed to suit war purposes; while the many bones that are found in caves, heaps and piles, indicate that many thousands fell in mortal combat then and there. Possibly they were old in the skilled arts of war at that day. Their great and powerful men, who should have been parents of the coming generations, were slain and destroyed and the conquered became the captives and slaves of the more powerful, with all opportunities for mental development suppressed. Other nations and tribes willingly entered the bloody fields of battle, with nothing to report but the death of the best physically formed men, and leaving the propagation of the race or races to be kept up by those who were left behind as unqualified to go into battle, for lack of strength of either body or mind.

This process of destroying the mentally and physically great has been kept up to the limits of our history's record. We have to go to schools about one-half of our time in order to cultivate and stimulate our mental energies sufficiently well, that we may follow the ordinary business pursuits of life.

MENTAL DWARFAGE.

Without worrying the patience of the reader any further, we will ask him if it is not reasonable that during all the past thousands of years, that men have fought over their gods and governments, has it not produced the mental dwarfage from the causes he has had to face? Our professional men are only imitators of one another. They must spend years in school because of a lack of native ability. This is our condition, and we must make the best we can of it. Most of our learned men, so-called, at the present day, stand upon heaps of mental rubbish. You seldom see in an editor's columns any evidence of mental greatness. He clips, quotes and sells his wisdom. He takes up some hobby, religious or scientific. He lauds his own religious views; his scientific ideas he wishes embalmed for the use of future generations. His law is *the* law. His medicine is God's pills, notwithstanding he is the laughing stock of all who know him. I want to be good to them. I expect to be good to them, as they are suffering from the effects of pre-natal causes, thrown upon them by their ancestors for thousands of years. By those causes they have been possibly wounded worse than I have, and I do not expect to spend any time in combats with mental dwarfs; political, religious, or scientific bigots. If I can successfully run my boat over the riffles of time, I shall credit it to good luck, not native ability, for I, too, feel what they should,—the deep plowings of mental dwarfage, that is the result of killing all the great and good men for ages.

CHAPTER XV.

OSTEOPATHIC TREATMENT.

Five Points—Visceral List—Care in Treating the Spinal Column—
Most Important Chapter—Perfect Drainage—A Natural Cure.

FIVE POINTS.

The five points of observation will cover easily the whole body, and
we cannot omit any one of them, and successfully examine any
disease of the system. Local injuries are, however, an exception to
this rule, and even a local hurt often causes general effect. Suppose a
fall should jar the lumbar vertebra, and push it at some articulation,
front, back, or laterally; say the lumbar, with one or two short ribs
turned down against the lumbar nerves with a prolapsed and
loosened diaphragm, pressing heavily on the abdominal aorta, vena
cava, and thoracic duct; have you not found cause to stop or derange
the circulation of blood in arteries, veins, lymphatics and all other
organs below diaphragm? Then heart trouble would be the natural
result. Fibroid tumors, painful monthlies, constipation, diabetis,
dyspepsia or any trouble of the system that could come from bad
blood would be natural results, because lymph is too old to be pure
when it enters the lungs for purifying. If blood or chyle is kept too
long below the diaphragm, it becomes diseased before it reaches the
lungs, and after renovation, but little good blood is left. Then the
dead matter is separated from blood and blown out at the lungs
while in vapor. Thus nutriment is not great enough to keep up
normal supply. In this stage the patient is low in flesh and feeble
generally, because of trouble with blood and chyle to pass normally
through the diaphragm.

VISCERAL LIST.

The failure of free action of blood produces general debility,
congestion, low types of fever, dropsy, constipation, tumefaction and
on to the whole list of visceral of diseases.

From this we are called to the pelvis. If the innominate bones are twisted on sacrum or are driven too high or too low, an injury to the sacral system of blood and nerves would be cause equal to congestion, inflammation of womb or bladder-diseases, with a crippled condition of all the spinal nerves. This would be cause enough to produce hysteria, and on to the whole list of diseases to spinal injuries. The Osteopath has great demands for his powers of reason when he considers the relation of diseases generally to the pelvis; and this knowledge he must have before his work can be attended with success.

As I said, five points comprise the fields in which the Osteopath must search. I have given you quite pointedly and at length, hints on spine and sacrum which cover the territory below the diaphragm. In conclusion I will simply refer you to the chest, neck and brain, and say, "let your search light ever shine bright on the brain." On it we must depend for power. About all nerves do run through the neck and branch off to supply both above and below, to do their parts in animal life, to the heart, brain and sum total of man and beast. Search faithfully for cause of diseases in head, neck, chest, spine and pelvis; for all organs, limbs and parts are directly related to and depend on these five localities to which I have just called your attention.

With your knowledge of anatomy, I am sure you can practice and be successful, and should be in all cases over which Osteopathy is supposed to preside.

CARE IN TREATING THE SPINAL CORD.

I want to offer you the facts, not advice, but pure and well sustained facts, the only witnesses that ever enter the courts of truth. A spinal cord is a fact; you see it—thus a fact. That which you can see, feel, hear, smell or taste is a fact, and the knowledge of the ability of any one fact to accomplish any one thing, how it accomplishes it and for what purpose, is a truth sought for in philosophy. The spinal cord is the present fact for consideration. You see it, you feel it, thus you have two facts with which you can start to obtain a knowledge of the use of this spinal cord. In it you have one common straight cylinder which is filled with an unknown substance, and by an unknown power wisely directed. It is wisely formed, located, and protected. It throws off branches which are wisely located. They have bundles, many and few; they are connected to their support, which is the brain, by a continuous cord in length and form to suit. After it has concluded throwing off branches at local places for special purposes, then like a flashlight, it throws off a bundle of branches called horse-tail plexus, *caudae equinae*, which simply signifies the many branches that convey fluids and influences to the extremities, to execute the vital work for which they are formed and located. While the laws of life and their procedure to execute and accomplish the work designed by nature for them to do, is mysterious and to the finite mind incomprehensible, you can only see what they do or perform, after the work is done and ready for your inspection.

HOW TO TREAT THE SPINAL COLUMN.

Now as we are dealing with the omnipresent nerve principle of animal life, I will tell you this one serious truth, and support it by the fact of observation. To treat the spine, and thereby irritate the spinal cord oftener than once or twice a week will cause the vital assimilation to be perverted, and become the death-producing excretor, by producing the abortion of the living molecules of life, before fully matured, while in the cellular system, which lies immediately under the lymphatics.

Your patients will linger long from the change of the nutrient ducts to throw off their dead matter into the excretories, which death was caused by the undue, or too many treatments of the spinal cord. If you will allow yourself to think for a moment, or think at all of the spinal cord being irritated, and what effect it will have on the uterus you will realize that I have told you a truth, and produced an array of facts to stand by that truth. Many of your patients are well six months before they are discharged. They are kept on hands because they are weak, and they are weak, because you keep them so from irritating the spinal cord. Throw off your goggles and receive the rays of the sunlight which forever stand in the bosom of reason.

MOST IMPORTANT CHAPTER OF ALL.

This is the most important chapter of this book, because at this point the engine of life is turned over to you as an engineer and by you it is expected to be wisely conducted on its journey.

Your responsibility here is doubled. Your first position is that of a master mechanic, who is capable of drawing plans and writing minutely a specification whereby the engineer may know what a well constructed machine is in every particular. He knows the parts and relations of both as constructor and operator, and you are supposed to be the foreman in the shop of repairs. The living person is the engine, nature the engineer, and you the master mechanic.

This being your position it is expected that you will carefully inspect all parts of the engines run into your repair shop, note all variations from the truly normal, and adjust from those variations as nearly as possible to the conditions of the true specimen that stands in the shop.

PERFECT DRAINAGE.

At this point it will be proper to suppose a case by way of illustration. Suppose by some accident the bones of the neck should be thrown at variance from the normal to a bend or twist. We may then expect inharmony in the circulation of the blood to the head and face with all the organs and glands above the neck. We will find imperfect supply of blood and other fluids to the head. We may expect swelling of head and face with local or general misery. Thus you have a cause for headache, dizziness, blindness, enlarged tonsils, sore tongue, loss of sight, hearing, memory, and on through the list of head diseases, all because of perverted circulation of the fluids of the brain proper of any local division. It is important to have perfect drainage, for without it, the good results from a treatment cannot be expected to follow your efforts to relieve diseases above the neck.

WHAT TREATING MEANS.

Here I want to emphasize that the word treat has but one meaning, that is to know you are right, and do your work accordingly. I will only hint, and would feel embarrassed to go any farther than to hint to you, the importance of an undisturbed condition of the five known kinds of nerves, namely: sensation, motion, nutrition, voluntary and involuntary, all of which you must labor to keep in perpetual harmony while treating any disease of the head, neck, chest, abdomen, pelvis, spine and limbs.

If you would allow yourself to reason at all, you must know that sensation must be normal and always on guard to give notice by local or general misery, of unnatural accumulation of the circulating fluids. Each set of nerves must be free to act and do their part. Your duty as a master mechanic is to know that the engine kept is in so perfect a condition that there will be no functional disturbance to any nerve, vein, or artery that supplies and governs the skin, the fascia, the muscle, the blood or any fluid that should freely circulate to sustain life and renovate the system from deposits that would cause what we call disease.

A NATURAL CURE.

Your Osteopathic knowledge has surely taught you, that with an intimate acquaintance with the nerve and blood supply, you can arrive at a knowledge of the hidden cause of disease, and conduct your treatment to a successful termination. This is not by your knowledge of chemistry, but by the absolute knowledge of what is in man. What is normal, and what abnormal, what is effect and how to find the cause. Do you ever suspect renal or bladder trouble without first receiving knowledge from your patient, that there is soreness and tenderness in the region of the kidneys at some point along the spine. By this knowledge you are invited to explore the spine for the purpose of ascertaining whether it is normal or not. If by your intimate acquaintance and observance of a normal spine you should detect an abnormal form although it be small, you are then admonished to look out for disease of kidneys, bladder or both, from the discovered cause for disturbance of the renal nerves by such displacement, or some slight variation from the normal in the articulation of the spine. If this is not worthy of your attention, your mind is surely too crude to observe those fine beginnings that lead to death. Your skill would be of little use in incipient cases of Bright's disease of the kidneys. Has not your acquaintance with the human body opened your mind's eye to observe that in the laboratory of the human body, the most wonderful chemical results are being accomplished every day, minute and hour of your life? Can that laboratory be running in good order and tolerate the forming of a gall or bladder stone? Does not the body generate acids, alkalies, substances and fluids necessary to wash out all impurities? If you think an unerring God has made all those necessary preparations, why not so assert, and stand upon that stone?

You cannot do otherwise, and not betray your ignorance to the thinking world. If in the human body you can find the most wonderful chemical laboratory mind can conceive of, why not give more of your time to that subject, that you may obtain a better understanding of its workings? Can you afford to treat your patients without such qualification? Is it not ignorance of the workings of this Divine law that has given birth to the foundationless nightmare that now prevails to such an alarming extent all over civilization, that a deadly drug will prove its efficacy in warding off disease in a better way than has been prescribed by the intelligent God, who has formulated and combined life, mind and matter in such a manner that it becomes the connecting link between a world of mind, and that element known as matter? Can a deep philosopher do otherwise than conclude that nature has placed in man all the qualities for his comfort and longevity? Or will he drink that which is deadly, and cast his vote for the crucifixion of knowledge?

CHAPTER XVI.

REASONING TESTS.

The Vermiform Appendix—Operating for Appendicitis—Expelling
Power of the Vermiform Appendix—Care Exercised in Making
Assertions—Reasoning Tests—A List of Unexplained Diseases—
Concluding Remarks.

THE VERMIFORM APPENDIX.

At the present time more than at any other period since the birth of
Christ, the medical and surgical world have centralized their minds
for the purpose of relieving locally inside, below the kidney of the
male or female, excruciating pain, which appears in both sexes in the
region above described.

From some cause, possibly justifiable, it has been decided to open
the human body and explore the region just below the right kidney
in search of the cause of this trouble. Such explorations have been
made upon the dead first. Small seeds and other substances have
been found in the vermiform appendix, which is a hollow tube over
an inch in length. These discoveries, as found in the dead subject,
have led to explorations in the same location in the living. In some of
the cases, though very few, seeds and other substances have been
found in the vermiform appendix, supposed to be the cause of local
or general inflammation of the appendix. Some have been
successfully removed, and permanent relief followed the operation.
These explorations and successes in finding substances in the
vermiform appendix, their removal, and successful recovery in some
cases, have led to what may properly be termed a hasty system of
diagnosis, and it has become very prevalent, and resorted to by the
physicians of many schools, under the impression that the
vermiform appendix is of no known use, and that the human being
is just as well off without it.

OPERATING FOR APPENDICITIS.

Therefore it is resolved, that as nothing positive is known of the trouble in the location above described, it is guessed that it is a disease of the vermiform appendix. Therefore they etherize and dissect down for the purpose of exploring, to ascertain if the guess is right or wrong. In the diagnosis this is a well-defined case of appendicitis; the surgeon's knife is driven through the quivering flesh in great eagerness in search of the vermiform appendix. The bowels are rolled over and around in search of the appendix. Sometimes some substances are found in it; but often to the chargrin of the exploring physician, it is found to be in a perfectly healthy and natural condition, and so seldom is it found impact with seeds or any substance whatever, that as a general rule it is a useless and dangerous experiment. The per cent of deaths caused by the knife and ether, and the permanently crippled, will justify the assertion that it would be far better for the human race if they lived and died in ignorance of appendicitis. A few genuine cases might die from that cause; but if the knife were the only known remedy, it were better that one should occasionally die than to continue this system, at least until the world recognizes a relief which is absolutely safe, without the loss of a drop of blood, that has for its foundation and philosophy a fact based upon the longitudinal contractile ability of the appendix itself, which is able to eject by its natural forces any substances that may by an unnatural move be forced into the appendix.[8]

EXPELLING POWER OF THE VERMIFORM APPENDIX.

To a philosopher such questions as this must arise: Has the appendix at its entrance a sphincter muscle similar in action to that of the rectum and œsophagus? Has it the power to contract and dilate?— contract and shorten in its length and eject all substances when the nerves are in a normal condition? And where is the nerve that failed to execute the expulsion of any substance that may enter the cavity of the appendix? Has God been so forgetful as to leave the appendix in such condition as to receive foreign bodies without preparing it by contraction or otherwise to throw out such substances? If He has He surely forgot part of His work. So reason has concluded for me, and on that line I have proceeded to operate for twenty-five years without pain or misery to the patient, and given permanent relief in all cases that have come to me. With the former diagnosis of doctors and surgeons that appendicitis was the malady, and the choice of relief was the knife or death, or possibly both, many such cases have come for Osteopathic treatment, and examination has revealed that in every case there has been previous injury to some set of spinal nerves, caused by jars, strains or falls. Every case of appendicitis, gall or renal stones can be traced to some such cause. These principles I have proclaimed and thought for twenty-five years.

CARE EXERCISED IN MAKING ASSERTIONS.

We should use much caution in our assertions that nature had made its work so complete in animal forms and furnished them with such wisely prepared principles that they could produce and administer remedies to suit, and not leave the body to find them. Should we so conclude and find by experiment that man is so arranged, and wisely furnished by deity as to ferret out disease, purify and keep the temple of life in ease and health; we must use great care when we assert such is not undeniably true up to the present. The opposite opinion has had full sway for twenty centuries at least, and man has by habit, long usage, and ignorance so adjusted his mind to submit to customs of the great past that should he try, without previous training, to reason and bring his mind to such altitude of thought of the greatness and wisdom of the infinite, he might become insane or fall back in a stupor, and exist only as a living mental blank in the great ocean of life, where beings dwell without minds to govern their actions. It would be a great calamity to have all the untrained minds shocked so seriously as to cause them to lose the mite of reason they now have, and be sent back once more to dwell in Darwin's protoplasm. I tell you there is danger, and we must be careful and show the people small stars, and but one at a time, till they can begin to reason and realize that God has done all that the wisest can attribute to Him.

REASONING TESTS.

There is but one method of reasoning. That method is by the laws governing the subject to be reasoned upon.

Reasoning is the action of the mind while hunting for truths.

THE ABDOMEN.

As we are about to camp close to the abdomen for a season of explorations and a more reasonable knowledge of its organs and their functions, we will search its geography first, and find its location on the body or globe of life. We find a boundary line established by the general surveyor, about the middle of the body, called the diaphragm. This line has a very strong wall or striated muscle that can and does dilate and contract to suit for breathing, and quantities of food that may be stored for a time in stomach and bowels for use. The abdomen is much longer than wide. In short, it is a house or shop built for manufacturing purposes. In it we find the machinery that produces rough blood or chyle, and sends it to heart and lungs to be finished to perfect living blood, to supply and sustain all the organs of this division. This diaphragm or wall has several openings through which blood and nutriment pass to and from abdomen to heart, lungs and brain. I want to draw your special attention to the fact that this diaphragm must be truly normal. It must be anchored and held in its true position without any variation, and in order that you shall fully understand what I mean, I will ask you to go with me mentally to all the ribs, beginning with the sternum, see attachments, follow across with a downward course to the attachments of this great muscular septum to the lower lumbar region, where the right crus receives a branch or strong muscle from the left side, and the left crus receives a muscle from the right which becomes one common muscle known as the left crus, the same of the right crus receiving a muscle or tendon from the left, which you will easily comprehend from examining descriptive cuts in Gray, Morris, Gerrish, or any well illustrated work of anatomy. You see at once a chance for constriction of the aorta by the muscles under which it passes, causing without doubt much of the disease known as palpitation of the heart, which is only a bouncing back of the blood that has been stopped at the crura. Farther away from the spine near the center of the diaphragm we find the return opening through this wall, provided to accommodate the vena cava. To the left a few inches below the vena cava we find another opening provided for the œsophagus and its nerves; like the aorta, it has two muscles of the diaphragm crossing directly between œsophagus and the aorta, in such shape as to be able to produce powerful prohibitory constriction to normal swallowing.

A LIST OF UNEXPLAINED DISEASES.

At this point I will draw your attention to what I consider is the cause of a whole list of hitherto unexplained diseases, which I think are only effects, caused by the blood and other fluids being prohibited from doing normal service by constrictions at the various openings of the diaphragm. Thus prohibition of free action of the thoracic duct would produce congestion of receptaculum chyli, because of not being able to discharge its contents as fast as received. Is it not reasonable to suppose a ligation of the thoracic duct at the diaphragm would retain this chyle until it would be diseased by age and fermentation, and be thrown off into the substances of other organs of the abdomen and set up new growths, such as enlargement of the uterus, ovaries, kidneys, liver, spleen, pancreas, omentum, lymphatics, cellular membranes, and all that is known as flesh and blood below the diaphragm? Have you not reason to explore and demand a deeper and more thorough anatomical knowledge of the diaphragm and its power to produce disease while in an abnormal condition, which can be caused by irritations, wounds or hurts, from the base of the brain to the coccyx? Remember this is an anatomical and philosophical question that will demand your attention to the mechanical formation, physiological action and the unobstructed privileges of fluids when prepared in the laboratory of nature, to be sent at once to their ordained destination, before such substances are diseased or dead with age. You must remember that you have been well drilled, or talked out of patience in the room of symptomatology and all you have learned is, something ails the kidneys, and are told their contents when analyzed are not normally pure urine. In urinalisis you are told "here is sugar," "here is fat," "here is iron," "here is pus," "here is albumen," and this is diabetis, this is Bright's disease, but no suggestion is handed to the student's mind to make him know that these numerous variations from normal urine are simply effects, and the diaphragm has caused all the trouble, by first being irritated from hurts, by ribs falling, spinal strains, wounds and on from the coccyx to the base of the brain. Symptomatology is very wide and wise in putting this and that together and giving it names, but fails to give the cause of all these abdominal lesions. Never for once has it said or intimated that the diaphragm is prolapsed by misplaced ribs to which it is attached, or that it is diseased by hurts of spine and nerves above its own location. Allow yourself to think of the universality of the distribution of the superior cervical ganglion and other nerves which are of such great importance that I will by permission insert in the last chapter of this book a description of that great system of the sympathetic nerves by Dr. Wm. Smith, whose superior knowledge of anatomy makes him eminently qualified to describe the location and uses of this great sympathetic system of the nerves of life.

CONCLUDING REMARKS.

As you read his able essay remember there are four other sets of nerves equal to, and just as important in their divisions of life, which are the motor, nutrient, voluntary and involuntary. All of which you as an engineer must know, and by proper adjustment of the body give them unlimited power to perform their separate and united parts in sustaining life and health. Now as I have tried to place into your hands a compass, flag and chain that will lead you from effect to cause of disease in any part or organ of the whole abdomen I hope that many mysteries which have hung over your mental horizon will pass away, and give you abiding truths, placed upon the everlasting rock of cause and effect. You have so little use for old symptomatology as an Irishman has for a cork when the bottle is empty. Osteopathy is knowledge, or it is nothing.

CHAPTER XVII.

OBSTETRICS.

Overloading—Similarity of Stomach and Womb—Births—
Preparation for Delivery—Caution—Lasceration Need Not Occur—
Care of Cord—Severing Cord—Putting on Belly Band—Delivery of
Afterbirth—Preparing for Mother's Comfort—Post-Delivery
Hemorrhage—Treatment for—Food for Mother—Treatment for Sore
Breast.

OVERLOADING.

When in the course of human events and actions of life, a woman
disregards the laws of nature to such an extent as to overload the
stomach beyond its powers and limits; or another way to present the
thought, we will say, if you fill the stomach so full as to occupy all
space, or so much of the space as to cripple the laws of digestion and
retain the food, the decomposition sets up an irritation of the nerves
of mucous membrane to such a degree as to cause sickness and
vomiting, or any other method of disgorging the stomach, which is
the natural process to unload an overloaded vessel. When the nerves
cannot take up nutrition, they will then take up destruction and
other elements which are detrimental to the process of nutrition, and
there is no other process for relief but to unload. The loading that has
been deposited in the stomach was for the purpose of sustaining a
being. The stomach itself is a sack. When filled to its greatest
capacity, it irritates all the surroundings, and in return they irritate
the stomach. Thus it unloads naturally for relief. Now we wish to
treat of another vessel similar in size, similar in all its actions, which
receives nourishment for a being, which nourishment is contained in
the blood, and conveyed from the channels commonly known as
uterine arteries. To all intents and purposes this nourishment is
taken there to sustain animal life, after having constructed the
machinery then it appropriates the blood to the growth and existence
of a human being. One is the womb, the other the stomach. The
placenta in the womb is provided with all the machinery necessary
to the preparation of blood, such as is used for all purposes in

141

forming and developing a child. Which is the stomach? Which is the womb? and what is the difference? Both receive and distribute nourishment to sustain animal life. Both get sick, both vomit when irritated and discharge their loading by the natural law of "throw up" and "throw down." Now note the difference and govern yourselves accordingly. One is mid-wifery, or treatment of the lower stomach during gestation and delivery. The other is the upper stomach that takes coarser material and refines the unrefined substances, keeps the outer man in form and being; the other contains the inner man or child, and by the law of ejection, when it becomes an irritant, it is thrown out by the nerves that govern the muscles of ejection.

BIRTHS.

To illustrate: I will say, just as long as digestion and assimilation keep in harmony and the mother generates good blood in abundance, the child grows, and by nature the womb is willing to let the work of building the body of the child go on indefinitely; but nature has placed all the functions of animal life under laws that are absolute and must be obeyed. We by reason are asked to note the similarity of the stomach and the womb, as both receive and pass nutriment to a body for assimilation and growth. When a stomach gets overloaded, sickness begins, as digestion and assimilation has stopped, then the decaying matter is taken up by the terminal nerves, and conveyed to the solar plexus, and causes the nerves of ejection, to throw the dying matter out of the stomach which is above. Try your reason and see the stomach below sicken and unload its burden. Is this sickness natural and wisely caused? If this is not the philosophy of mid-wifery what is? As soon as a being takes possession of its room, the commissary of supplies begins to furnish rations for that being, who has to build for itself a dwelling place. The house must be built strictly to the letter of the specifiction. Much bone and flesh must be put into the house of life, and some of all elements known to the chemist, must be used and wisely blended to give strength; also all material to be used in the house must be exact in form and given strength equal to all forces, that may be necessary to execute the hard and continued labors of the machinery that may be used in all transactions and motions of mind and body. Now we must go to the manufacturing chief, and have him through the quartermaster deliver and keep a full supply of all kinds of material for the work, and when the engine is done, put it on an inclined plane and cut the stay-chains and let it run out of the shop. Be careful and not let the engine deface nor tear the door as it comes out. A question is asked: On what road does the quarter-master send the supplies? As there is but one system over which an engine can bring supplies, we will call that road the uterine system of arteries. The mechanic reports that he will open the door of this great shop of manufacturing, and let it roll out the engine by the power and methods prepared to run out finished work. First you see a door open because the lock is taken off by a key that opens all mysteries; and the great ropes that have been far inferior to the force of resistance, that has held the door shut, are all sufficient in power. By getting sick, muscles become convulsed to rigidity of great strength with force enough to push the new engine of life out into open space easily, by nature's team that never fails to obey orders to deliver all goods intrusted to its care.

PREPARATION FOR DELIVERY.

A student of mid-wifery can only learn a few general principles, before he gets into the field of experience. Actual contact with labor teaches him that much that he has read and had told to him by professors of mid-wifery in the lectures, is of but little use to him at the bedside. What he needs to know is, what he will have to do after he gets there. He must know the form and size of the bones of a woman, how large a hole the three bones of the pelvis make, for the reason that the child's head will soon come through that hole. He must know a normal head cannot come through a pelvis that has been crushed in so much as to bring the pubis within one and one-half to two and one-half inches of the sacrum. He must examine and know, and do this soon after he is called, for the reason, that he will have to use instruments in such deformities, and may wish the counsel of an older and more experienced doctor. And this precaution will give him time to be ready for any emergency.

But more than ninety per cent of all cases are of a very simple nature. The mother is warned by pains in back and womb, coming and repeating at intervals of one-half hour to less time. When by the finger the doctor can tell the mouth of the womb has opened to the size of a quarter or half dollar, he then may know that labor will soon start in good earnest, and at this time it is well to call for a twine, cut two strings about a foot long, to tie around the navel cord.

CAUTION.

The first duty of the obstetrician is to carefully examine the bones of the pelvis and spine of the mother, to ascertain if they are normal in shape and position. If there is any doubt about the spine and pelvis being in good condition for the passage of the head, through the bones, and you find pelvic deformity enough to prohibit the passage of the head, notify the parties of the danger in the case at once, and that you do not wish to take the responsibility alone, as it may require instruments to deliver the child, as there is danger of death to the child and mother also, but less danger to the mother than to the child. Now you have done that which is a safeguard against all trouble following criminal ignorance.

I will give you a condensed rule of procedure in all normal cases of obstetrics. With index finger, examine os uteri; if closed and only backache, have patient turn on right side, and press hand on abdomen above pelvis, and gently press or lift belly up just enough to allow blood to pass down and up pelvis and limbs. Relax all nerves of the pelvis at pubes.

SECOND EXAMINATION.

Caution: Wait a few hours; examine os again. If still closed and no periodical pains are present, you are safe to leave case in the hands of the nurse, instructed to send for you if regular pains return at intervals. On your return, explore os again, if found to open as large as a dime, you are by this notified that labor has begun its work of delivery. You now place patient on her back, propped to an easy angle of near thirty degrees, with rubber blanket in place. After you find os, dilated to nearly the size of a dollar, then relax nerves at pubes. Soon you will find in mouth of womb an egg-shaped pouch of water, which you must not press with fingers till very late in labor, for fear of stopping labor for perhaps many hours. Remember the head can and does turn in pelvis to suit the easiest passage through the bones, while in the fluids of the amniotic sack. Now, as you know why not to rupture sack and spill fluids, you are prepared to proceed to other duties, which are to prevent rupture of perineum. Place the left hand on the belly, about two inches above symphesis and push the soft parts down with the left hand; support the perineum with the right hand until head passes over. This is necessary to prevent rupture of perineum.

LASCERATION NEED NOT OCCUR.

If you follow this law of nature, lasceration may occur in one out of a thousand cases, and you will be to blame for that one, and may be censured for criminal ignorance. Now you have conducted head safely through pelvis and vagina to the world. You will find pains stop right short off for about a minute, which is the time to learn whether the navel cord is wrapped around the child's neck.

CARE OF CORD.

If it is found all around the neck once or more, you must slip finger down neck and loosen cord to let blood pass through the cord till next pain comes, in order to ward off asphyxia of child.

When pain comes, gently pull child's head down toward the bed. There is no danger of hurting the perineum now since the head has passed the soft parts. At this time the danger is suffocation of child. Never draw child too far away from mother's birth place by force, as you may tear navel string from the child and cause it to bleed to death. If you value the life of the child, then you must be careful not to place the navel end of the string in any danger of being torn off. Now you have made a good job for both mother and child so far. The child is in the world; and you want to show the mother a living baby for her labor and suffering of the past nine months. The baby is born and the mother is not torn, but the baby has not yet cried. Turn it on its side, face down, run your finger in its mouth and draw out all fluids, thick or thin, to let the breath pass to the lungs. Then blow cold breath on its face and breast to cause its lungs to act.

SEVERING CORD.

Baby cries, all is safe now. Baby is born safely and cries nicely, but still has cord fastened to afterbirth. It has no further use for cord, as life does not depend upon blood from the afterbirth any longer. Take the cord about three inches from the child's belly, between thumb and finger, and strip towards child to push bowels out of the cord if there should be any in it, as a safeguard for bowels, then tie a strong string around cord, first three inches from child's belly, second, four inches; take the cord in your hand and look what you are doing. If baby's hand should fall back to cord, you might cut off one or two fingers, or wound the hand or arm very seriously. Cut cord between the two ties just made on navel string. Look out for your scissors; pass the child over to the nurse to be washed and dressed, while you deliver the afterbirth from pelvis or womb.

PUTTING ON BELLY BAND.

When the child's shirt is on, cut a hole the size of your thumb in a doubled piece of cloth, five inches long by four wide, put the hole two inches from one end, and run the cord through the hole. Lay the cloth across the child's belly, then fold the cloth lengthwise over the cord, which must lie across the child so it will not stretch cord by handling or straightening child out. Now you are ready to finish the delivery of the afterbirth. You have a plug of soft and tender flesh to get out of the womb and vagina.

DELIVERY OF AFTERBIRTH.

As the afterbirth has been grown tight to the womb during all the days of mother's pregnancy, and furnished all the blood to build and keep the child alive in the womb for nine months, it has done all it can do for the child, and is now ready to leave the womb.

You are there to assist it to get out of the place it has occupied so long. You must begin first to rotate or roll the placenta first one way and then another, up, down and across the vagina, by gently pulling the cord. Look out or you will pull the cord loose from the placenta; then you will have made your first blunder,—no cord to pull placenta with, and the mother bleeding and faint from loss of blood. Now is the time and place to save life. Pass your hand forward into the soft parts to get your fingers behind the placenta; now give a rolling pull and bring it out with the hand. You will find it an easy matter to get your hand into the vagina and womb after the birth of the child. Get all the placenta out, then take a wad of cloth or rags as large as the child's head, and press it under the cross bone of the pelvis; push the cloth under and up, so as to completely plug the pelvis. Now pull the hair gently over the symphesis, which will cause the womb to contract by irritation.

PREPARING FOR MOTHER'S COMFORT.

All is now done but to provide for the mother's comfort, which is your next duty. Draw her chemise down her back and legs until it is straight, then with safety pins, pin the chemise on inner side of thighs so that the chemise will go around both thighs separately. Now you have the shirt fast to keep it from sliding upwards, and you are ready to make a band of the chemise to support the womb and abdomen. Bring the chemise tightly together for two or three inches above the pelvis to form a band. Previous to pinning, draw the lump (womb) you feel above symphesis, up, then pin, and the belt you have made of the chemise will support the womb. All is safe now, but you must not leave for two hours. You may have delivered a feeble woman, who may flood to death after delivery of the child, if you do not leave her safe. I have in mind one case who flooded all of two quarts at a single dash. The first symptom was a pain in the head.

POST-DELIVERY HEMORRHAGE.

I know of only two causes that would produce hemorrhage or bleeding after the child is delivered. One is when the afterbirth

147

(placenta), is separated from its attachment to the womb and still retained in the womb or vagina, or when a part is separated and still lies in the womb, that retention of placenta prevents the natural circular contraction of the womb, to close on itself and retain it, with force enough to prevent the further discharge of blood, would give a chance for a continued stream. Then should the patient bleed profusely after the placenta has been removed, another cause would be in pulling away the afterbirth, as part of the upper portion of the womb may be pulled to an inverted position, which would be like a hat if you press the top down with the hand. Then there is a chance for leakage because of this unnatural fold made in the womb.

TREATMENT FOR.

My method of relief is to insert the hand, and with back of fingers smooth out all folds. Before you draw the right hand from the womb place left hand on abdomen, catch the womb between the thumb and finger and withdraw hand. With the left hand pull the hair above symphesis or scratch the flesh just above across the region of the symphesis, just enough to make an irritation. After the hand is out of vagina pass a small bundle of cloths as far under the symphesis as would be necessary to hold everything up, then fasten chemise; beginning at symphesis draw it tight for about two inches above symphesis and with strong pins fasten it. Be sure you keep garment tight by pulling down between limbs. The coarser the chemise the better, as you want to make a strong bandage at that point so as not to push the womb down into the pelvis. If the patient's general health is fairly good let her tell you what she wants to eat, and go and get it. Let her diet be after her usual custom. You must remember she has just left the condition of a full abdomen. Lace her up, fill her up and make her comfortable for six hours; then change her bedding.

FOOD FOR MOTHER.

Remember this, if you stop digestion on her for some hours with teas, soups and shadows to eat, you carry her to the condition where it would be dangerous to give her a hearty meal. My experience and custom for forty years has been crowned with good success. I never lost a case in confinement. I have universally told the cook to give her plenty to eat.

TREATMENT FOR SORE BREAST.

If she begins to have fever followed by chilly sensations, with swelling of one or both breasts, I relieve that by laying her arm ranging with her body. Let some one hold the arm down to the bed, then I place both of my hands under the arm, pull it up with considerable force till I get it as high or higher than normal position of the shoulder. Then pull her shoulder straight out from the body a fairly good pull, then pull the arm up on a straight line with the face, and be sure that you have let loose the axillary and mammary veins, nerve and artery, which have been cramped by pulling the arm down during delivery. No breast should become caked in the hands of an Osteopath. Do not bother about the bowels for two or three days. It may be necessary to use the catheter if the water should fail to pass off after inhibiting the pubic system. This is straight mid-wifery and will guide you through at least in ninety per cent of the cases you will meet in normally formed women.

Right here I wish to say one word: I think it is very wrong to teach, talk and spend so much time with pictures, cuts, talks and lectures, and hold up constantly to the view of the student, births coming from the worst imaginable deformities and call that a knowledge of mid-wifery. It is normal mid-wifery you want to know and be well-skilled in. The abnormal formations are few and far between, and when a case of that kind does appear, it is your knowledge of the normal that guides you through the variations. You will very likely never find two abnormals presenting the same form of bone. As this is intended to only present to the student natural delivery I will let the subject drop with one word about the sore tongue of the mother. Adjust her neck, relieve constrictor and all other muscles that would impede any blood vessel that should drain the mouth and tongue. Remember this, that a horse that is always hunting bugars never finds a smooth road.

CHAPTER XVIII.

CONVULSIONS.

Old Phrases—Results of Stoppage of Fluids—Old Theory of Fits—
What the Real Cause may be—Listen for the Cause—What is a Fit—
Sensory System Demanding Nourishment—The Causes—The
Remedy—Dislocation of Atlas and of Four Upper Ribs.

OLD PHRASES.

As old phrases that have long been in use as names for the various
diseases have almost grown to the degree of disgust, I laid them
aside and have been trying and have succeeded in unfolding natural
laws to a better understanding, which do and should be our guide
and action in treating all diseases that mar the peace and happiness
of the human race by misery and death. By such old systems with
their foolish and unreliable suggestions, of how to guide the doctor
in treating diseases which have proven unworthy of respect, if merit
is to be our rule of the weights and measures of intelligence. I have
become so disgusted with such verbiage with the sense that follows
the pens that have written treatise on disease, that I have concluded
to do like Adam of old, give names that may appear novel to the
reader when I wish to draw the attention of the student who is trying
to obtain a knowledge of the mysteries hitherto unsolved and
unexplained. We have panned and washed by their suggestions and
have obtained no gold. There are two very large and powerful rivers
passing their fluids in opposite directions over a territory that I will
call the Klondike of life. This territory is bounded on the east by a
great wall, which according to the old books has been called the
diaphragm, through which comes forth a great river of life that
spreads all over the plains of the anterior lumbar region. On that
plain we find a great system of perfect irrigation of cities, villages,
and fertile soils of life.

RESULT OF STOPPAGE OF FLUIDS.

This region of country covers one of the greatest and most fertile fields of life producing elements, and places them on the thoroughfares, and sends them back over the great central railroad, the thoracic duct, from lymphatics of the whole abdomen, to the heart and lungs to be converted into a higher order of living matter. When finished it is called blood, to sustain its own machinery, and all other machines of the body, giving rise to the mental question: "What would be the effect produced to life and health, if we should cut off, dam up or suspend the flowing of the aorta as it descends close by the vena cava and thoracic duct as they return with contents through the diaphragm on their journey to the heart and lungs for manufacture and finish. And after having supplied the plain, what would be the effect if the vena cava and its system of drainage, and the thoracic duct should be dammed up so that chyle and blood could not be carried to the heart and lungs for renewal, purification, and finish. How much thought would be required to see that by stopping the arterial flow or that of the vena cava an irritating and famishing condition would ensue, with congested veins, lymphatics and all organs of the abdomen, to that condition called fermentation, congestion and inflammation, which in time is thrown off by sloughing away the substances of the lymphatics of the whole abdominal system of glands that belong to a liver, a kidney, the uterus and the bowels, to the condition that has long since been a mystery, and called typhoid fever, dysentery, bilious fever, periodical spasms, and on through the whole list of general and special diseases of winter and summer. I would advise the practicing Osteopath to do some very careful panning up and down the rivers of this Klondike, for if you fail to find gold, and much of it, you had better spend the remainder of your life where reason dwelleth not. Ever remembering that ignorance of the geography and customs of this country is the wet powder of success."

OLD THEORY OF FITS.

We often see a woman or man afflicted with fits or falling sickness which the doctor has failed to cure. What is a fit? For want of a better knowledge we have an established theory that "hysteria" is purely her imagination and as we must respect old theories, we will call it a fit of meanness. This is what we have had for breakfast, dinner and supper and we are asked to respect such trash because of the "established theories."

We are instructed by the universal "all" of the graduates of various medical schools to call her a criminal and proceed to punish her with a wet towel, well twisted, and administered freely—more comprehensively expressed by the term "spanker" and "spank her" very much—late from Scotland with all Europe, and schools in America, except the American School of Osteopathy, which recommends to "wallop" and "wallop" very freely the empty headed schools and theories that have no more sense than to torture a sick person and do so to disguise their ignorance of the cause of her disease, which is shown by the spasmodic effect that has been named by a little book of guess work, generally called and universally known as symptomatology.

WHAT THE REAL CAUSE MAY BE.

Not a single author has hinted or in any way intimated that the cause of her disease is a failure of the passing of the blood, chyle and other substances to and from the abdomen to nourish and renovate the abdominal viscera caused by a prolapsed diaphragm, which would cause resistance to the passing of the aorta, through which passes the arterial blood through the crura, and the vena cava that returns the venous blood, and through which crura the chyle is conducted from the receptaculum chyli before decomposition by fermentation sets up.

LISTEN FOR THE CAUSE.

The afflicted is intoxicated. Here is where she gets a poisonous alcohol and will never be relieved permanently until the "wet towel" of reason has slapped on both sides of the attending physician's head, so he can hear the squeezing and rattling of regurgitation, and straining and creaking of the fluids in their effort to pass through that great and strong towel called the diaphragm. Until he learns this

I would apply the wet towel of reason to the doctor, for fear he becomes lukewarm in his studies and gives his patient a hypodermic injection of morphine, which is the advice as given at the last council of medical men who practice "old established" theories rather than be honest enough to say: "The woman is sick and I know it, but I do not know the cause of her trouble."

WHAT IS A FIT?

What is a fit? If God's judgment is to be respected a fit is the life-saving step and move, perfectly natural, perfectly reasonable, and should be so respected and received as divinely wise, because on that natural action which is produced on the constrictor nerves first, then the muscles, nerves, veins and arteries with all their centers. It appears at this time that the vital fluids have all been used up, or consumed, by the sensory system, and in order to be temporarily replenished, this convulsion shows its natural use by squeezing vital fluids from all parts of the body to nourish and sustain the sensory, which has been emptied by mental and vital action, until death is inevitable without this convulsing element to supply the sensory system, though it may be but a short time.

SENSORY SYSTEM DEMANDING NOURISHMENT.

The oftener the fits come, the oftener the nutrient system of the sensory cries aloud in its own, though unmistakable language, that it must have nourishment, that it may run the machinery of life, or it must give up the ghost and die. In this dire extremity and struggle for life, it has asked the motor system to suspend its action, use its power and squeeze out of any part of the whole body though it be the brain itself, a few drops of cerebro-spinal fluid, or anything higher or lower, so it may live.

Those of you acquainted with the fertile fields of the Klondike referred to, will be enabled to furnish the sensory system with such nutriment, as will not make it necessary to appeal to you through the language used by the unconscious convulsions with all their horrible contortions.

THE CAUSES.

Thus you surely see with the microscope of reason that the sensory nerves must be constantly nourished, and that all nutriment for the nerves must be obtained from the abdomen, though its propelling force should come directly from the brain.

THE REMEDY.

The nerve courses from the brain must be unobstructed from the cerebrum, cerebellum, the medulla oblongata, and on through the whole spinal cord; with a normal neck, a normal back, and normal ribs, which to an Osteopath means careful work, with power to know, and mind to reason that the work is done wisely to a finish. I hope that with these suggestions you will go on with the investigation to a satisfactory degree of success.

DISLOCATION OF THE FOUR UPPER RIBS.

I wish to insert a short paragraph on a few effects following a down, front, and outer dislocation of the four upper ribs of either side. We have been familiar with asthma, goitre, pen-paralysis, shaking palsy, spasms, and heart diseases of various kinds. We have been as familiar with the existence of those abnormal variations as we are of the rising and the setting of the sun. Our best philosophers on diseases and causes have elaborately written and published their conclusions, and the world has carefully perused with deep interest, what they have said of all the diseases above named, also diseases of the lung, and to-day we are by them left in total darkness as to the cause of the above named diseases, also fits, insanity, loss of voice, brachial agitans, and many other diseases of the chest, neck and head. As the field is open and clear for any philosopher to establish his point of observation, note and report what he observes, I will avail myself of this opportunity, and say in a very few words, I have found no one of the diseases above indicated to have an existence without some variation of the first few of the upper ribs of the chest. With this I will leave farther exploration in the hands of other persons; and await the report of their observations pro and con.

CHAPTER XIX.

CONCLUDING REMARKS.

Thoughts for Consideration—Offering a New Philosophy—
Lymphatics and Fascia—A Satisfactory Experiment—Natural
Washing Out.

THOUGHTS FOR CONSIDERATION.

"Let us not forget the assembling of ourselves together." Whether this quotation applies to us or not, as an Osteopath I will venture to say that the honored dead, and the honest living intelligent healers of all schools, and all systems of trying to relieve our race from disease and suffering, so far as I have been able to ascertain, have been forced to guess how to proceed when they enter the "sick room" for want of a philosophical system of procedure. We have collected together many or few symptoms, named the disease, opened the battle, and on our side have met the enemy and fought bravely all battles very much the same way. I have spent one-half of a century in the field trying the many methods of attacks; and used the best arms and ammunition to date, and designed to do the greatest good. For twenty years or more I was content to be governed by the opinions and customs of older and more experienced physicians. I gave the disease its proper name. I gave the medicine as taught and practiced, but was not satisfied that the line of procedure was philosophically correct.

OFFERING A NEW PHILOSOPHY.

I believe at the present time I am fully prepared to say I can offer you a more rational philosophy of what should be the physician's first object, when called to repair a vessel that has become unseaworthy by accumulated barnacles, and is placed upon the dry dock for restoration to that condition called seaworthy, again. I believe this philosophy will sustain the strongest minds in the conclusion that our first and wisest step to successfully combat all diseases would be to inhibit first the nerves of the lymphatics, then produce muscular constricture and cause them to unload their diseased contents, and keep them unloading until renovation is absolutely complete; leaving the lymphatics in a purely healthy state, and keep them in this condition at any period of the disease. I have long since been of the opinion that if we could keep all impurities from accumulating in the lymphatics, and never allow them to become overloaded, we would have no such diseases as bilious fever, typhoid, mountain fever, malaria, pneumonia, flux, heart disease, brain disease, fits, insanity and on to the whole list of climatic troubles, and the troubles with the changes of winter and summer.

LYMPHATICS AND FASCIA.

I have thought for many years that the lymphatics and cellular system of the fascia, of the brain, the lungs, and the heart throughout the whole system of blood supply, do get filled up with impure and unhealthy fluids, long before any disease makes its appearance, and that the procedure of changes known as fermentation, with its electromagnetic disturbances, were the cause of at least ninety per cent of the diseases that we labor to relieve by some chemical preparation called drugs. When I was fully satisfied that we were liable to do more harm than good with such remedies, I began to hunt for more reasonable methods to relieve the system of its poisonous gases and fluids, through the excretory system of the lymphatics and other channels, through which we had hoped to renovate and purify the system.

A SATISFACTORY EXPERIMENT.

For twenty-five years I have tried to balance myself, divert my mind from all previous methods and see if I could not get more directly to the lymphatic system of nerves, and cause the millions of vessels known to exist in the body to begin to unload their contents and continue that action until all impurities were discharged by way of the bowels, lungs, kidneys and porous system.

NATURAL WASHING OUT.

At the conclusion of this philosophy I will endeavor to explain just how nature has provided to ward off diseases, by washing out before fermentation should set up in the lymphatics, from being received and retained the length of time, that destructive chemical changes would begin its work of converting elements into gas and discharging them from the system as unsuitable for nutriment. In order to avoid this calamity we are met with two important thoughts, one of the power of the nerves of the lymphatics to dilate and contract, also that of fascia and muscle, to dilate or constrict with great force when necessary to eject substances from gland, cell, muscle and fascia. Thus we see a cell loaded to fullness by secretion which it cannot do without; open-mouthed vessels through which it receives this fluid. Then again the system of cellular sphincters must dilate and contract in order to retain the fluids in those cell-like parts of the body. Now we are at the point when ready for use in other parts of the system, those sphincters must temporarily give away, that the gland may relax and dilate. Then the universal principle of constriction throughout the whole body can discharge the contents of the lymphatics of all divisions of the body, which is surely the normal condition. Let the lymphatics always receive and discharge naturally. If so we have no substance detained long enough to produce fermentation, fever, sickness and death.

I think this thought has been presented plainly enough to be fully understood and practiced by the reader, if an Osteopath.

CHAPTER XX.

THE SUPERIOR CERVICAL GANGLION.

With what it has Communication—Its Position—One of its Functions—Stimulation or Inhibition—Results Produced.

WITH WHAT IT HAS COMMUNICATION.

Every ganglion on the great chain of the sympathetic nerve has special and important functions, but upon the superior cervical falls the greatest burden of responsibility. This ganglion has communication with a greater number of nerves and organs than any other; is in direct communication with three cranial and four cervical nerves, indirectly with four more cranial nerves, and enters, by its branches into the formation of a large number of plexuses. Through this ganglion it is that much Osteopathic work is done, and the purpose of this brief paper is to point out some of the many effects which may be produced by its stimulation or inhibition.

ITS POSITION.

Anatomically we know that the superior cervical ganglion is situated in relation to the transverse processes of the upper three cervical vertebrae. It gives off branches which communicate directly with the vagus, glosso-pharyngeal and hypoglossal nerves; another branch, the ascending, passes into the carotid canal and enters into the formation of the carotid and cavernous plexuses; other branches pass to the pharynx, and a branch enters the formation of the cardiac plexuses. From the carotid and cavernous plexuses pass many nerves, only a few of which need special mention; one unites with the great superficial petrosal to form the Vidian nerve which goes to *Meckel's* ganglion, branches pass to the Gasserian ganglion, while we have others passing to the third, fourth, the ophthalmic division of the fifth and the sixth nerve, also we have derived from the nerve the sympathetic root of the lenticular ganglion.

ONE OF ITS FUNCTIONS.

Physiologically we know that one of the special functions of the sympathetic nervous system is to control the tone of non-striate muscular tissue, and that we have filaments distributed from the sympathetic system in the muscular wall of every blood vessel, duct and organ throughout the body. We also know that the sympathetic is the accelerator nerve of the heart, being opposed in its action by the vagus which, is inhibitory; further, that the vagus is constant in its brake-like action, while the sympathetic only acts when stimulated either directly or reflexly. While the vagus is inhibitory to the heart it is motor to the lungs. Nerve force is not generated in the sympathetic system; the cerebro-spinal nerve force is conveyed to the ganglia by the rami communicantes and in the ganglia is transformed into sympathetic nerve force. We might compare the ganglia to electrical transformers. Such being the case it is not difficult to see that if the superior cervical ganglion receives the nerve-force for transformation from the upper four cervical nerves and we can prevent, or lessen, the passage of nerve-force from the spinal cord through those nerves to the ganglion, that we will, to a corresponding degree, lessen the amount of sympathetic nerve-force transformed in the ganglion and transmitted from it by its branches.

STIMULATION OR INHIBITION.

We can produce stimulation or inhibition of a nerve at will; press suddenly and with a little violence upon the ulnar nerve where it lies in relation with the internal condyle of the humerus and we will find a manifestation of its physiological action, evidenced by a sense of pain in the ulnar and radial sides of the fifth finger and the ulnar side of the fourth, together with contraction of the muscles supplied by that nerve. But if our pressure be less intense and more prolonged we will inhibit the nerve and produce a sense of numbness in the same area together with temporary loss of muscular control.

Osteopaths well understand how to produce either stimulation or inhibition of the ganglia by way of the nerves passing to them from the spinal cord, and the results of such inhibition or stimulation in any sympathetic area can be prophesied readily by anyone who has read with attention what I have written; for instance, in the case of inhibition in the region of the nerves supplying the superior cervical ganglion with nerve force, we will find, first, throughout the area of distribution of the branches of this ganglion a relaxation of the vascular walls. This will be marked by two indications, first, the skin will become flushed and moist; second salivary secretion and lachrymal secretion will be increased. Second, the vagus is now allowed full sway, and we will find slowing of the heartbeat. It is well known that pressure over the seat of the first spinal nerve for a very brief period of time will control a congestive headache; the pressure in such case is made only for so long time as to produce stimulation of the sympathetic to greater activity, when we will attain a vaso-constrictor action, lessen the volume of blood in the cranial cavity and so abolish the headache. The arteries of the body may be divided into three groups, the large, the medium-sized and the small; in the first of these we find little muscular tissue and much elastic; in the second they exist in about equal proportions, while in the small arteries we find much muscular tissue and little elastic. As a consequence it is upon the smaller arteries that the sympathetic system has its greatest effect. As we dilate the smaller arteries and slow the heart action, it follows that we reduce the blood pressure, as we reduce blood pressure we reduce temperature, and within a very few minutes after the commencement of this inhibitory pressure on the upper four cervical nerves we will find in the large majority of cases, the capillaries over the entire surface of the body flushed, this being accompanied by a fall in the pulse rate and a marked diminution of the temperature. Indirectly at the same time we produce an effect upon the lungs; as we lessen blood pressure and the frequency of the heart action we find in accordance with the physiological rule an alteration in the respiration, it becomes slower and deeper. Arguing along these lines, and applying similar reasoning to each of the branches of this ganglion, anyone can trace out the many subsidiary results which may be expected from either stimulation of the rami communicantes nerves distributed to it, or their inhibition. Exactly similar rulings will find their prompt proof with regard to any other of the ganglia of the sympathetic system. We will find corresponding results in the cases of the thoracic ganglia which form by their branches the pulmonic plexuses; we get the same results from the splanchnic ganglia; while in the lumbar region we find that we have a ready means of control of the vascular system in the lower abdomen and pelvis. Much, very much, is still to be learned concerning the sympathetic nervous system, and all such increase in knowledge can come in one way only, clinical observation of Osteopathic treatment.

WILLIAM SMITH,
L. R. C. P. and S., (EDIN.), D. O.

THE END.

FOOTNOTES

[1] Explore: (1) To seek for or after: to strive to attain by search; to look wisely and carefully for; to search through or into; to penetrate or range over for discovery; to examine thoroughly; as, to explore new countries or seas; to explore the depths of science; "hidden frauds (to) explore." —WEBSTER.

[2] Chambers.

[3] "The secretion of the external auditory meatus, mixed with the secretion of the neighboring glands or ceruminous glands, forms the well known ear-wax or cerumen. The secretion in this place contains a reddish pigment of a bitterish sweet taste, the composition of which has not been investigated." American Text-Book of Physiology.

[4] Chambers.

[5] DISEASE. 1. "Lack of ease. 2. An alteration in the state of the body, or some of its organs, interrupting or disturbing the performance of the vital functions and causing or threatening pain and weakness; malady; affection; illness; sickness; disease; disorder." —Webster's International Dictionary.

[6] What has the student gained by reading the above definition of this standard author and representative of present medical attainment but a labored effort to explain what he does not know.

[7] Very true, if treated by the medicine man.

[8] My first Osteopathic treatment for appendicitis was in 1877, at which time I operated on a Mr. Surratt and gave permanent relief. During the early eighties I treated and permanently cured Mrs Emily Pickler of Kirksville, mother of our representative, S. M. Pickler, and mother of ex-congressman John A. Pickler of South Dakota. The infirmary has had bad cases of appendicitis probably running up into hundreds without failing to relieve and cure a single case. The ability of the appendix to receive and discharge foreign substances is taught in the American School of Osteopathy and is successfully

practiced by its diplomates. In the case of Mr. Surratt I found lateral twist of lumbar bones; I adjusted spine, lifted bowels, and he got well. When I was called to Mrs. Pickler she had been put on light diet, by the surgeon, preparatory to the knife. She soon recovered under my treatment without any surgical operation and is alive and well to this date.

A. T. Still's Table or Device,

That He Has Constructed For

The Use of The Operator, The Ease And Comfort of The Patient.

It is a welcome success and does away with the lubberly old tables. It gives ease and support to all classes of patients. By its use the patient can sit in a chair or on a stool and feel at perfect ease during all treatments, then the operator gets results and is not tired to death when he has treated a patient; knows and feels that there has been some good done.

The asthmatic knows he has gotten help because pain has left his chest and he breathes as with new lungs; he knows he is helped more by one treatment while sitting on a chair with his body easy and at rest in the cushioned swinging device than he would or has received by the best skill on any table. Then the operator says, "Thank fortune, I am not worn out, and know I have gotten every bone to the place it belongs, and I know I have given satisfactory relief because my patients say so."

I think to an operator this device is his best friend. With it well understood he can do as much work as three good operators can do on the old tables. Remember this device does no part of the treatment but places the patient to your convenience while you do the work.

I feel as I am the discoverer of the device, that I know its needs and feel free to advise pupils.

The device will cost you $25 only.

A. T. STILL,
Founder.

Lightning Source UK Ltd.
Milton Keynes UK
175916UK00001B/198/P

9 781409 957546